Evaluation in Dementia Care

Evaluation in Dementia Care

Edited by Anthea Innes and Louise McCabe

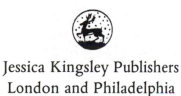

Jessica Kingsley Publishers
London and Philadelphia

First published in 2007
by Jessica Kingsley Publishers
116 Pentonville Road
London N1 9JB, UK
and
400 Market Street, Suite 400
Philadelphia, PA 19106, USA

www.jkp.com

Copyright © Jessica Kingsley Publishers 2007

The right of the contributors to be identified as authors of this work has been asserted by them in accordance with the Copyright, Designs and Patents Act 1988.

Library of Congress Cataloging in Publication Data
Evaluation in dementia care / edited by Anthea Innes and Louise
McCabe. -- 1st American pbk. ed.
    p. ; cm.
    Includes bibliographical references and index.
    ISBN-13: 978-1-84310-429-2 (pbk.)
    ISBN-10: 1-84310-429-6 (pbk.)
    1. Dementia--Patients--Care. 2. Dementia--Patients--Services for.
3. Dementia--Treatment--Evaluation.   I. Innes, Anthea.
II. McCabe, Louise.
    [DNLM: 1. Dementia--nursing. 2. Long-Term Care--methods.
3. Health Services Research--methods. 4. Outcome and Process
Assessment (Health Care)--methods. 5. Research Design.
WY 152 E92 2007]
    RC521.E93 2007
    616.8'3--dc22

                                                        2006019503

British Library Cataloguing in Publication Data
A CIP catalogue record for this book is available from the British Library

ISBN-13: 978 1 84310 429 2
ISBN-10: 1 84310 429 6

Printed and bound in Great Britain by
Athenaeum Press, Gateshead, Tyne and Wear

Contents

Acknowledgements

We would like to thank Charlie Murphy for his input to the early development of this book, for his ideas about structuring the book and the topics that the book should cover. We would also like to thank Alison Dawson for her skilful contribution to putting the book together and careful checking of the manuscript.

PART ONE

Contexts of Evaluating Dementia Care

Chapter 1

What is Evaluation?

Anthea Innes and Louise McCabe

What do we mean by evaluation?

Evaluation is something that we do on a daily basis; we may have to evaluate what would be the best clothes to wear for today's weather, weighing up the likelihood of a need for an umbrella. We may also have to evaluate the time we have to reach a destination, and decide whether to walk, drive or catch a bus. There are a number of texts devoted to the topic of evaluation; however, there is no consensus on a specific definition of 'evaluation'. The term 'evaluation' is widely used by authors when reporting on so-called 'evaluations', yet Patton (1982) has demonstrated that only half of the 170 reports he reviewed could properly justify the use of the word 'evaluation'. Within the literature devoted to the exploration of evaluation there is a common focus, that of evaluation as a process of learning, making decisions or gathering information.

For example, evaluation has been conceptualized as a learning process which involves 'considering failures and weaknesses...reflection and critical analysis, recommendations and further action' (Moriarty 2002, p.8). There is also a focus on evaluation as a contributor to change or what Øvretveit has called 'evaluation for action' (1998, p.15) where as a result of the evaluation someone should be able to act or make a more informed decision. Evaluation has also been described as a practice for gathering information (Patton 1982) which takes the form of what Øvretveit (1998) has termed a descriptive evaluation design.

Evaluation can also encapsulate the learning process, decision-making process and information-gathering process. For example, Herman, Morris and Fitz-Gibbon (1987) set out a conceptual framework to understand evaluation. They suggest that the underlying framework for evaluation is a:

> ...belief that evaluation can play an integral role in improving program operations and contribute to enlightened policy making at federal, state, local, agency and corporate levels...well-conceived, well-designed and thoughtfully analysed evaluations can provide valuable insights into how programs are operating, the extent to which they are serving their intended beneficiaries, their strengths and weaknesses, their cost-effectiveness and potentially productive directions for the future. (p.8)

They suggest that evaluation can help to set priorities, guide the allocation of resources, facilitate the modification and refinement of programme structures and activities and signal the deployment of personnel and resources. Similarly Øvretveit (1998) suggests that 'evaluation is making a comparative assessment of the value of the evaluated or intervention, using systematically collected and analysed data in order to decide how to act' (p.9). Thus an outcome for evaluation is the availability of information to help those commissioning the evaluation to make decisions.

How do we do evaluation?

Rossi, Lipsey and Freeman (2004) suggest that there are three forms an evaluation may take: the independent evaluation; a participatory or collaborative evaluation; and an empowerment evaluation (p.51). An independent evaluation is when an external party undertakes the evaluation (discussed by Lechner in Chapter 3), collaborative evaluations involve multiple stakeholders (Chapters 6 and 10 provide specific examples of this approach), while an empowerment evaluation has an aim to enable those being evaluated to have some form of control and/or say in the programme evaluated (discussed by Murphy in Chapter 12).

This is developed further by Øvretveit (1998) who suggests that evaluation can use six broad designs:

1. descriptive; this may involve describing a service, the features of an intervention or an implementation process

2. audit; where a care setting is compared against a standard set of criteria

3. before–after; compares a setting before and after an intervention occurs

4. comparative-experimentalist; compares the before and after states of two different interventions in two different settings

5. randomized controlled experimental; comparison of defined before and after state between two groups, one allocated an intervention and one a placebo

6. intervention to an organization which has two forms – impact for providers and impact for service users (pp.54–65); compares the before and after states of providers or service users following the introduction of an intervention.

Øvretveit's evaluation design may be carried out in an independent, collaborative or empowering way as described by Rossi *et al.* (2004). Thus the design of an evaluation can adopt a particular starting point, that of collaboration, empowerment or 'fact finding'. An important point stressed by Øvretveit (1998, pp.33–35) is that evaluations should be systematic in their approach, no matter what design is used and what methods are adopted. Patton defines the practice of evaluation as:

> ...the systematic collection of information about the activities, characteristics and outcomes of programs, personnel and products for use by specific people to reduce uncertainties, improve effectiveness and make decisions with regard to what these programs, personnel and products are doing and affecting. (1982, p.15)

The need for a flexible approach for the conduct of evaluation is widely recognized (Herman *et al.* 1987; Patton 2002; Rossi *et al.* 2004). The emphasis on techniques often dichotomized as qualitative or quantitative in their approach is evident with Herman *et al.* (1987) placing emphasis on measuring, while Patton (2002) has a primary concern with qualitative methods of enquiry. However, a common feature of the evaluation literature is recognition of the need for and support for an eclectic approach to evaluation and the need to employ techniques suited to that which is to be evaluated. That is to take the starting point of – which methods are most appropriate to the question we are seeking to answer?

Why evaluate dementia care?

The reason for evaluating dementia care will vary according to those 'stakeholders' who are involved in the evaluation process. Although not writing specifically about dementia care, Rossi *et al.* (2004, pp.48–49) suggest a range of evaluation stakeholders who are likely to be involved in a dementia care evaluation:

- policy makers and decision makers
- programme sponsors
- evaluation sponsors
- target participants (people with dementia, carers)
- programme managers
- programme staff.

Competitors, contextual stakeholders (organizations, groups and individuals in the vicinity of the programme to be evaluated) and the evaluation and research community are other potential groups of stakeholders (Rossi *et al.* 2004, p.49). Those conducting an evaluation need to be aware of the views, concerns and agendas of those stakeholders who may be involved in or have an active interest in the conduct and findings from any evaluation.

There are, however, likely to be two over-arching rationales behind dementia care evaluations:

- To assess the outcomes (intended or otherwise) of a service or care intervention for the service user, care worker or organization.
- To monitor the impact of a specified change to service delivery for the service user and/or service provider.

These may be guided by a desire of the service provider to secure further funding to maintain an existing service which is time and resource limited, or to provide evidence that the service provided is 'good' and thus have a rationale for promoting it, increasing costs and extending provision. Thus it is important that evaluators have a clear understanding of the reason(s) for undertaking an evaluation prior to beginning the process of information gathering.

Why focus on evaluation in dementia care?

The growing plethora of policy directives with explicit expectations of standards of care (for example, Department of Health 2002; Scottish Executive 2004; Welsh Assembly Government 2004) give rise to a policy context where care providers are expected to provide certain levels of care (see Chapter 4 for further discussion). In addition there has been a practice concern to improve care practice reflected in the common parlance of 'person-centred care' and the need to focus on the person with dementia (Kitwood 1997), alongside the increase in expectations that users' views should be taken into account when planning, developing and evaluating services (Wilkinson 2002). Despite the growing focus on standards of care, person-centred approaches and seeking the views of people with dementia there is not a large literature on evaluation and dementia. While there are accounts of dementia care evaluations (Barnett 2000; Cantley *et al.* 2000; Murphy 2000), these are not devoted to 'how to do' evaluation. This book is not a 'how to do it' guide but it does provide insights into how to approach evaluating dementia care.

Thus contributors do not revisit an entire evaluation (results, recommendations and so on) in which they have been involved, rather they use the particular evaluation(s) to focus on aspects of the evaluation process. Therefore, lessons are drawn out on aspects such as setting up an evaluation; measurement and analysis; challenges in feeding back results; and implementation of recommendations. Consequently the book offers readers a mixture of both the practical/descriptive account of an evaluation and educational/reflective accounts.

This book covers the topic of evaluation from three angles. First, different levels of evaluation, for example the programme level, service level and intervention level; second, different settings, for example in the community and in long stay care; and third, reflections on different aspects of the evaluation process.

The structure of the book

The first section, 'Contexts of Evaluating Dementia Care', provides an overview of the context for evaluating dementia care. Cantley (Chapter 2) provides an overview of the difficulties in approaching the evaluation of dementia care. She discusses six key problems in dementia care evaluation: pursuing the experimentalist ideal, developing alternative methodologies, measuring outcomes, involving service users, handling practical issues and working ethically. Such problems are revisited and reflected upon by contributors in subsequent chapters, for example Wijk considers evaluating dementia care, within the experimentalist ideal, while Innes and Kelly consider how to build on 'in vogue' methods to evaluate dementia care, and measuring outcomes is of concern to Bowes, Wijk, and Gibson, Haight and Michel. Practical issues are touched on by all chapter contributors, while involving service users is discussed by Tyrrell, Christie and Murphy. Working ethically is considered explicitly by Christie and Murphy but is an implicit concern throughout this book. Thus Cantley provides a contextual overview for those seeking to evaluate dementia care which is discussed throughout the book.

Lechner (Chapter 3) provides insights into the pros and cons of evaluating your own workplace and evaluating the workplace of other dementia care workers. She highlights the tensions that can arise in both internal and external evaluation situations. McCabe (Chapter 4) sets evaluation within a policy context and reminds us that evaluations are often a result of policy requirements as are actions that may be required following the findings of an evaluation.

The second section focuses on practicalities of conducting dementia care evaluations with each author providing personal reflections on the process of conducting an evaluation, either in day care, care in the community or long stay care. Bowes (Chapter 5) discusses the approach of 'pragmatic evaluation' to technological interventions, highlighting the importance of ethical conduct and establishing a good communicative process with service users. She also cautions that the full costs and benefits of providing technology for people with dementia need to be explored and understood in order to provide a full overview of the impact and outcome of technology for service users. Wijk (Chapter 6) considers evaluating the environment where dementia care occurs. She discusses how the impact of design features can be evaluated using resident-related outcome measures and staff-related outcome measures as part of a discovery process about what design features enhance the quality of life for people with dementia.

Gibson, Haight and Michel (Chapter 7) describe the evaluation of a life review and life storybook project carried out in a variety of residential settings. The outcomes of an intervention provided by caregivers after limited training and supportive supervision included positive individualized interactions with people with dementia. Innes and Kelly (Chapter 8) consider evaluating long stay dementia services and the role of Dementia Care Mapping (DCM) in this process. Based on their experiences they discuss strengths and limitations of the method when trying to evaluate a care setting. They suggest that DCM can be useful as part of a 'tool kit' of techniques to help evaluate dementia care in a holistic way mirroring the philosophy of holistic dementia care. Kirkevold (Chapter 9) draws on an evaluation of long stay care and considers a common intervention in care settings, that of medication and who benefits from the concealment of medication. Following a discussion about how medications may be administered, covertly in food and beverages, he reflects on how such practice can be evaluated. Tyrrell (Chapter 10) provides an example of the challenges in evaluating choices made by the person with dementia in decision making, an issue of increasing topicality. She reflects on methodological challenges inherent in involving people with dementia in evaluating decision making processes about their care. She demonstrates that despite such challenges it is possible to find out what people with dementia think about decisions made about their care options. There are three themes which flow between chapters in Part Two: user involvement, how methods 'fit' with the topic to be evaluated, and ongoing challenges of evaluating dementia care.

The final section develops these themes as future challenges facing those evaluating dementia care. The ethics of evaluation are reviewed by Christie (Chapter 11) reminding us of the need for consent, confidentiality and adhering to professional codes of conduct. Christie alerts the reader to ethical questions that should be considered when planning an evaluation, for example why the evaluation is being undertaken and how the findings will be used. She sets out criteria for conducting an ethical evaluation which are limited to participants with dementia, for example ensuring that participants have knowledge about the evaluation, that they are aware that they can choose not to participate and that they can complain if they are not happy with the process. Christie also highlights some specific issues those conducting an evaluation of dementia care must consider. These include providing an ongoing process of providing information and maintaining the consent of participants, ensuring legal safeguards are adhered to and allowing sufficient time to hear the voice of participants. Murphy (Chapter 12) reminds us of the need to include the views of service users in evaluation; he provides examples of how challenges can and have been overcome in the last decade and points the way to increases in user involvement in the future. He sets out three aspects of hearing users' views. First, practical and logistical considerations, such as establishing a relationship with the person with dementia and prioritizing this relationship over the asking of questions, modifying the questioning to follow a conversation approach and abandoning the questioning if necessary. Second, ethical considerations, echoing the points made by Christie (Chapter 11), about obtaining consent and also highlighting issues of interpretation of the words people with dementia use and avoiding tokenism. Third, how users' views fit into the context of evaluation, emphasizing the users' views of what is 'successful' rather than the evaluator or a professional's view about the experience of receiving the service or the aims of a service and other stakeholders' views about the impact of the service for the recipient.

Macijauskiene's account (Chapter 13) sets evaluation in the context of scarce resources and competing priorities in the provision of dementia care, particularly relevant with the global interest in dementia care. Finally McCabe and Innes (Chapter 14) provide a synopsis of the lessons that can be drawn from this book and how these could be applied in the future.

References

Barnett, E. (2000) *I Need to Be Me: Including the Person with Dementia in Designing and Delivering Care.* London: Jessica Kingsley Publishers.

Cantley, C., Smith, M., Clarke, C. and Stanley, D. (2000) *An Independent Supported Living House for People with Early Onset Dementia: Evaluation of a Dementia Care Initiative Project.* Newcastle upon Tyne: Dementia North.

Department of Health (2002) *NHS Framework for Older People.* London: Department of Health.

Herman, J.L., Morris, L.L. and Fitz-Gibbon, C.T. (1987) *Evaluator's Handbook.* Newbury Park: Sage.

Kitwood, T. (1997) *Dementia Reconsidered: The Person Comes First.* Buckingham: Open University Press.

Moriarty, G. (2002) *Sharing Practice: A Guide to Self-evaluation in the Context of Social Exclusion.* London: Arts Council England. www.newaudiences.org.uk/feature.php?news_20040701_3.

Murphy, C. (2000) *'Crackin' Lives': An Evaluation of a Life Story Book Project to Assist Patients from a Long-stay Psychiatric Hospital in their Move to Community Care Situations.* Stirling: DSDC.

Øvretveit, J. (1998) *Evaluating Health Interventions.* Buckingham: Open University Press.

Patton, M.Q. (1982) *Creative Evaluation.* London: Sage.

Patton, M.Q. (2002) *Qualitative Research and Evaluation Methods* (Third edition). Thousand Oaks: Sage.

Rossi, P.H., Lipsey, M.W. and Freeman, H.E. (2004) *Evaluation: A Systematic Approach.* Thousand Oaks: Sage.

Scottish Executive (2004) *National Care Standards.* www.scotland.gov.uk/topics/Health/care/17652/9325.

Welsh Assembly Government (2004) *National Minimum Standards for Domiciliary Care Agencies in Wales.* www.wales.gov.uk/subisocialpolicycarestandards/content/regulations/dom-care-wales-e.pdf.

Wilkinson, H. (2002) 'Including people with dementia in research: methods and motivations.' In H. Wilkinson (ed.) *The Perspectives of People with Dementia: Research Methods and Motivations.* London: Jessica Kingsley Publishers.

Chapter 2

Problems in Evaluating Dementia Care

Caroline Cantley

Let us consider the following questions:

- Is this new drug treatment for dementia effective?

- What has been the impact of introducing a new care planning system to providing care?

- Is this day care centre effective?

- Is setting up a specialist dementia team within home care a good way to manage our services?

- What has been the impact of the national initiative to promote better services for younger people with dementia?

- What has been the impact of the operation of continuing care charging policies in relation to people with dementia?

- How effective is the provision of support and information for people with early stage dementia individually compared with provision in groups?

- Is extra care housing a good alternative to care homes for people with dementia?

These are examples of the kind of questions that are frequently asked by service users, practitioners, managers, policy makers and researchers who are concerned with the provision and development of care for people with dementia. And they all have one feature in common. They are *evaluative* questions. And that should not surprise us. For questions of an evaluative nature lie at the heart of dementia studies, whether our interest is in the development of the field as an academic discipline or in the improvement of support for people with dementia and their carers.

However, questions of an evaluative nature are seldom easy questions to answer. They invariably present us with technical methodological problems and they are also complicated by the broader socio-political context of dementia care provision in which they arise. So in this chapter we shall consider some of the main problems in evaluating dementia care, bearing in mind throughout that the general socio-political context of health and social care must be understood, for it is often socio-political pressures that are significant in generating evaluative questions in the first place.

These are some of the pressures that I am referring to:

- Moves to make health service provision, and increasingly social services provision, more evidence-based.

- The strong emphasis on performance management of services and requirements for services to demonstrate their worth.

- Changing assumptions about the role of service users and carers with increasing emphasis on involving them in making choices about the services that they receive.

And more specifically related to dementia care:

- The commercial interests of drug companies in developing new treatments.

- Political fears about the resource consequences of growth in the number of people with dementia and in demand for services.

- Developments in the way we understand dementia and the experience of living with dementia.

- The recent growth in innovation and development in practice and service provision.

- The stronger voice for service users, for example through the growth and development of organizations such as the Alzheimer's Society and Alzheimer Scotland.

These socio-political, and economic, factors are instrumental not only in bringing evaluation to the fore in dementia care but also in affecting how evaluation is approached conceptually, methodologically, practically, politically and ethically. In this chapter I therefore consider six main problems in dementia care evaluation: pursuing the experimentalist ideal; developing alternative methodologies; measuring outcomes; involving service users and carers; handling practical issues; and working ethically.

Pursuing the experimentalist ideal

I noted above that one of the drivers of evaluation in dementia care is the requirement to demonstrate a sound evidence base. Within biomedicine, the approach to producing such evidence is grounded in positivism, rationality and objectivity, with the 'gold standard' being the scientific experiment or randomized controlled trial (RCT).

Since medicine, nursing, clinical psychology and other allied health professions are highly influential within dementia care, it is hardly surprising that experimental, or quasi-experimental, approaches to evaluation are widely used and regarded by many in dementia care as the ideal. Although much less widely adopted in social research, the experimental tradition is still important. For example, Challis *et al.* (1997) provide a good illustration of a significant study that used a quasi-experimental design to assess the impact of an intensive case management service for people with dementia. However, the successful implementation of experimental evaluations to produce a sound evidence base in dementia care is not without problems.

The controversy surrounding the National Institute for Health and Clinical Excellence (NIHCE) review of its original guidance (NICE 2001) on the use of anti-dementia drugs provides a good example of the problems. Even in an area like this, where the RCT methodology is largely unquestioned, there can be substantial difficulties. The review of evidence of the effectiveness of anti-dementia drugs undertaken for the Health

Technology Assessment Programme (Loveman *et al.* 2004) noted a wide range of methodological limitations amongst the studies undertaken. These included: the quality of reporting, length of follow-up, attrition (i.e. drop out of study participants), limitations regarding dose comparison, different treatment populations between studies, issues regarding the representativeness of sample populations, different outcome measures between studies, and difficulty in knowing what the recorded changes on some measures mean.

Central to the debates over the revision of the NICE guidance was the issue that the evaluation of effectiveness at population level does not tell us anything about the impact of the drugs on an individual (see Loveman *et al.* 2004). Thus a key basis on which clinical and service user representatives sought to influence the NICE guidance was that some people benefit more from these drugs than others (NIHCE 2005).

We also see the difficulties of achieving the experimental ideal in relation to psychosocial therapies. Systematic reviews of RCTs undertaken in the following areas note caution about findings or inability to draw conclusions:

- The effectiveness of cognitive training for early stage Alzheimer's disease (Clare *et al.* 2005).

- Aromatherapy for dementia (Thorgrimsen *et al.* 2005).

- Light therapy for managing sleep, behaviour and mood disturbances in dementia (Forbes *et al.* 2005).

- Music therapy for people with dementia (Vink *et al.* 2005).

- Reminiscence therapy for dementia (Woods *et al.* 2005).

- Validation therapy (Neal and Briggs 2005).

- Snoezelen for dementia (Chung and Lai 2005).

The reviewers' reservations were due variously to methodological limitations and difficulties, and to differences in findings, in the different RCT studies that met the criteria to be included in the review.

The response to such problems is typically a call for more and better RCTs. For example one review concluded:

> Whilst four suitable randomized controlled trials looking at reminiscence therapy for dementia were found, several were very small studies, or were of relatively low quality, and each examined different types of reminiscence work. Although there are a number of promising indications, in view of the limited number and quality of studies, the variation in types of reminiscence work reported and the variation in results between studies, the review highlights the need for more and better designed trials so that more robust conclusions may be drawn. (Woods *et al.* 2005)

In relation to broader service evaluations, the problems of the experimentalist ideal are compounded. An early study in which I was involved in looking at the problems of evaluation happened to take place in the context of what was essentially a leading edge dementia service of its time, then called a 'psychogeriatric day hospital'.

We identified a range of difficulties of pursuing the experimentalist ideal (Smith and Cantley 1985) in general and as they applied in this service context. Thus, in this service, and more generally in service evaluations:

- the controls of the clinical trial are seldom available

- the nature of the programme to be evaluated is often not clearly established at the start of the evaluation and, especially with new programmes, it often evolves over time

- the objectives of the programme are often not clearly stated

- different 'stakeholders' often have different views about what a programme should be trying to achieve and about what constitutes success.

Gibson, Haight and Michel in Chapter 7 explore in detail an example where an RCT type approach was taken to evaluate a reminiscence therapy for people with dementia.

The broader recognition of problems such as these, and related theoretical debates, have led on to the development of a range of alternative evaluation methodologies and it is to this that I now turn.

Developing alternative methodologies

Evaluation needs to be understood in the context of broader conceptualizations of research and the nature of knowledge.[1] A range of evaluation methodologies have been developed, based on different theoretical frameworks, that are critical of the positivist assumptions underpinning the scientific method and experimentalist ideal. These methodologies draw on different philosophical traditions but essentially all employ qualitative research methods and emphasize the importance of subjective experience and the ways in which we variously perceive, interpret, construct and talk about reality in social context. These approaches include: illuminative evaluation (Parlett and Hamilton 1977); pluralistic evaluation (Smith and Cantley 1985); fourth generation evaluation (Guba and Lincoln 1989); and critical evaluation (Everitt and Hardiker 1996). Relatively few studies in dementia care provide exemplars of these different approaches, but for a detailed account of the development of pluralistic evaluation in the context of dementia care see Smith and Cantley (1985) and for an account of the use of fourth generation methodology in dementia care see Pritchard and Dewing (2001).

Qualitative service evaluation methodologies adopt different approaches to eliciting the views of the people involved in the service, to understanding their perspectives and to taking into account those perspectives in reaching evaluative conclusions. This type of methodology generally sits comfortably alongside notions of personhood and social models of dementia (see Bond and Corner 2001). The benefits of this type of methodology tend to be accepted more readily by evaluators and dementia care practitioners who have their primary knowledge base in the social sciences than by those whose knowledge base is primarily biomedical.

There are a number of overviews and critiques of qualitative evaluation methodologies and their underpinning theoretical assumptions (see for example Murphy *et al.* 1998 and Spencer *et al.* 2003). For, as with positivism and the scientific ideal, there are significant limitations as well

---

1   The literature in these areas is vast and it is not my purpose to review that here. Bond and Corner (2001) provide a useful overview of the issues as they relate to research on dementia.

as strengths in qualitative research methods and evaluation methodologies. So, it is important that we are prepared to scrutinize qualitative evaluations as rigorously as those undertaken within the positivist tradition. For this purpose, Spencer *et al.* (2003) provide a framework for assessing qualitative evaluations in social research. The framework includes 18 appraisal questions based on the four principles that studies should be: contributory, defensible in design, rigorous in conduct, and credible in claim. Thus studies should be assessed as to whether they: play a part in advancing wider knowledge or understanding; have a research strategy appropriate to the questions being asked; are systematic and transparent in data collection, analysis and interpretation; and make claims that are well argued on the basis of the data generated.

Debates about the relative merits and limitations of scientific, experimental and quantitative approaches versus qualitative, subjectivist approaches have often become polarized with evaluators adhering strongly to one or other tradition. There have been some attempts to step outside these debates to develop other methodologies (for example realistic evaluation described by Pawson and Tilley 1997). At the level of evaluation practice, in dementia care as in other fields, many studies draw on different methodologies and employ a combination of qualitative and quantitative methods. This combination of methodologies and methods may result from pragmatism on the part of evaluators. However, in dementia care it can also be a deliberate and very constructive strategy, based on bringing an inter-disciplinary perspective to the evaluation of services which often are themselves founded on a range of assumptions (for example biomedical, psychosocial, social disability) about the nature of dementia and dementia care.

The challenge for any evaluator is to ensure that the approach chosen is appropriate for the questions being asked and rigorous in relation to the use to which the findings will be put. Evaluators need to resist being pressurized into a particular stance by those funding the evaluation or by other stakeholders who may have vested professional or other interests in the adoption of a particular approach.

Measuring outcomes

In the current health and social care policy and management context, there is much concern that service organizations should be able to demonstrate, and preferably quantify, successful outcomes. Outcome measurement is a crucial component of experimental and other quantitative evaluation approaches. In addition it is often a component of designs that combine quantitative and qualitative methodologies. Moriarty and Webb (2000) for example describe a multi-dimensional approach to evaluating community care support for people with dementia and their carers. Data collection, which was by interview at two time points 11 months apart, involved open and closed questions and a variety of standardized measures.

One of the greatest challenges in evaluation of dementia care is the development of appropriate outcome measures (Downs 1997). There are difficulties in doing so even in areas such as drug treatments where outcome measurement at first sight might appear straightforward. For example, Traynor, Pritchard and Dewing (2004) criticize the use of RCTs in evaluating the effectiveness of drug treatments for over-relying on a limited range of outcome measures relating mainly to cognition, activities of daily living and global functioning. These measures, they argue, are pre-determined by professionals and are based on limited appreciation of how measured changes relate to the day-to-day lived experience of people with dementia and their families.

Problems with determining outcomes are also evident in broader service evaluations. For example, Richards *et al.* (2003) in a study of services for people experiencing the early stages of dementia found that while there were no differences in cognition at 12-month follow-up between groups receiving different services (a memory clinic, CMHT and specialist day hospital), there were differences in frequency of day-to-day problems and caregiver mood. The authors suggest that:

> ...whilst standard measures of cognition may be of interest to researchers and perhaps to clinicians, more realistic measures of psychosocial disability such as day-to-day problems and caregiver experience over time, are at least of equal, if not greater importance to families. (p.8)

More generally, Moriarty and Webb (2000) note that evaluation of community support for people with dementia had largely used the outcome measure of admission to long-term care (see Downs 1997). They also note that the appropriateness of this measure had been challenged on the basis that effective services may not lead to change on this count and that this measure gives little indication of service impact on users and carers.

One significant step in developing our understanding of appropriate outcomes in dementia care was reported by Bamford and Bruce (2000). They demonstrated that it was possible, through group discussions with people with dementia, to identify their views about the outcomes of community care that are important to them. The outcomes they identified included the following quality of life outcomes:

- access to social contact and company
- having a sense of social integration
- access to meaningful activity and stimulation
- maximizing a sense of autonomy
- maintaining a sense of personal identity
- feeling safe and secure
- feeling financially secure
- being personally clean and comfortable
- living in a clean and comfortable environment.

We look now in more detail at how quality of life measurement has been approached in dementia care research.

Quality of life

Quality of life measurement, or more specifically health-related quality of life (HRQoL) measurement, has become a cornerstone of evidence-based health care. HRQoL is a multi-dimensional concept covering physical, psychological and social aspects of quality of life as they relate to health or health services. Measures of quality of life are frequently used as a means of evaluating the impact of treatment or services. However, quality of life is a multi-faceted and complex concept and there are many difficulties associated with its measurement (Bond and Corner 2004).

Many standardized instruments have been developed to measure quality of life, often using multi-item rating scales. Until recently, researchers approached the measurement of quality of life of people with dementia largely through use of proxy ratings or observation (for example using Dementia Care Mapping, discussed below). However, there are problems with relying on proxies. Novella *et al.* (2001) found that there was poor agreement between the assessments of quality of life by people with mild to moderate dementia and the assessments of proxies. Agreement was higher in relation to directly observable functions (for example physical abilities) and lower in relation to more subjective areas. Smith *et al.* (2005b) also found differences between the ways in which people with dementia and carers report HRQoL. They found that the difficulties in carers' reporting of HRQoL for people with dementia included being unable to avoid talking about their own reactions, and focusing on functional ability rather than how this impacted on HRQoL.

One response to the problems with HRQoL measurement has been to develop a conceptual framework based on the views of people with dementia and their carers. Thus Smith *et al.* (2005b), based on interviews with people with dementia and carers, have identified a wide range of aspects of quality of life that they grouped into five domains of quality of life that were important to people: daily activities and looking after yourself; health and well-being; cognitive functioning; social relationships; and self-concept. They suggest that the domain of self-concept appears to be unique to dementia. They note that further work is needed to clarify concepts of HRQoL with people with more severe dementia (see Thompson 2005).

Smith *et al.* (2005a) report on a new measure, DEMQOL, which takes seriously the incorporation of the subjective experience of people with dementia. This has both self-reported and proxy-reported measures and they recommend that both sets of measures are used together as they give 'different but complementary perspectives' (p.iii).

No discussion of quality of life assessment in dementia care would be complete without mention of Dementia Care Mapping (DCM), probably the best-known and probably most widely used dementia-specific quality measurement approach. DCM is an observational tool with foundations in the theoretical perspectives on person-centred care developed by Kitwood (1997). It is designed for use in group care facilities. An observer, known as a 'mapper', records at intervals, and against a structured coding frame, their assessment of the individual's well-being or ill-being and categories of behaviour, as well as instances of 'positive events' or 'personal detractions' that occur. DCM has been used in the evaluation of various interventions on the lives of people with dementia, in practice development evaluations where the data from repeated evaluations are used to inform a continuous quality improvement cycle, and in multi-method evaluations of single facilities or services (Brooker 2005).

Based on a wide-ranging review of the literature on its use, Brooker (2005) assesses the strengths of DCM as follows:

> …DCM seems to be suited to smaller scale within-subjects or group comparison intervention evaluations, given that it appears to demonstrate discrimination on a variety of interventions. In multi-method qualitative designs, DCM appears to enrich the data derived from proxy and service-user interviews and focus groups. DCM provides an opportunity to represent a reflection on what could be the viewpoint of service users who are unable to participate fully in interviews. (p.16)

As ever, no tool is without limitations. Bamford and Bruce (2002) identify the following for DCM: it can only be used in communal settings; the empirical basis for its underlying assumptions about well-being are limited and these assumptions may not be valid for everyone with dementia; and it relies on the evaluators' interpretations and does not give a direct voice to people with dementia.

The following comment by Brooker (2005), about why DCM has been so widely adopted by services, sits well with the starting premise of this chapter about the importance of the socio-political context of services in shaping evaluation:

> DCM provides a shared language and focus across professional disciplines, care staff and management teams. It is seen as a valid measure by frontline staff as well as those responsible for managing and commissioning care. It also provides a shared language between practitioners and

researchers. DCM holds a unique position in relation to quality of life in dementia care, being both an evaluative instrument and a vehicle for practice development in person-centred care. Many of the intervention evaluations cited above have been undertaken because DCM has given practitioners a way of trying to evaluate their practice. (Brooker 2005, p.17)

For an applied discussion of the use of DCM see Chapter 8.

Some broader considerations

There are some strong critics of outcome and quality of life measurement. Bond and Corner (2004) believe that:

> ...the move towards generic measures of outcome in evaluation research devalues the contributions of individual factors. Its use may simplify statistical analysis...but it masks the contribution of specific aspects of quality of life that may be important in the context of the intervention. Frequently in evaluation research this kind of outcome discriminates between experimental and non-experimental groups but we are often left trying to understand what it is that the outcome represents in the life world of study participants. (p.109)

They argue that quality of life should not be used as a 'formalized psychometric concept' but is best used as a concept that helps us to discuss and understand people's subjective accounts of their well-being.

We certainly need to be careful about focusing too much on outcomes, as other matters are also important to service users and carers. For example, Bamford and Bruce (2000) found that, as well as the quality of life outcomes listed above, the following aspects of service processes were important to people with dementia using community care support services:

- having a say in services
- feeling valued and respected
- being treated as an individual
- being able to relate to other service users.

The advice of Nocon and Qureshi (1996) on community care outcomes more generally is also apt in drawing attention to the broader context of outcomes in dementia care evaluation. They suggest that in constructing measures it is important to:

- take into account professional expertise and research-based knowledge
- understand the context in which the measures are to be used
- recognize and incorporate the perspectives of different stakeholders
- attach importance to the views of service users and carers.

In the next section, I consider more broadly the issue of involving service users and carers.

Involving service users and carers

Until recently service users were primarily perceived as passive subjects of research and evaluation. However, as the movement towards greater 'user involvement' in services has grown, so too has a movement towards involving service users in research and evaluation. In so far as service evaluations in dementia care obtained service user perspectives, they focused 'almost exclusively' on carers (Downs 1997). Although Dening and Lawton (1998) suggest that carers' perspectives had not been used much in evaluating old age psychiatry services, there has been a much longer tradition in social research of seeking the views of carers of people with dementia (for example, Levin, Sinclair and Gorbach 1983; Smith and Cantley 1985). See Chapter 12 for an in-depth discussion.

Often in dementia care evaluation carers are asked to contribute 'proxy' views for people with dementia. However, it is well established that carers' experiences and perceptions of service provision can be significantly different from those of the people for whom they are caring (Aggarwal *et al.* 2003; Bamford and Bruce 2000; Gilliard 2001; Hancock *et al.* 2003). Bamford and Bruce (2000) attributed differences in views to carers having difficulty identifying the outcomes of services for people with dementia, in part because they often got limited direct feedback from the person themselves, but also because they often had limited contact with the services. They also suggested that carers were reluctant to criticize services and that carers could not easily distinguish their own views from those of the person with dementia. Partly in response to these difficulties, there have been calls (for example Cheston, Bender and Byatt 2000; Stalker, Gilliard and Downs 1999) for more directly obtaining the perspectives of people with dementia in service evaluations.

Recently there has been a shift in practice with much more attention being paid, at least in more qualitative evaluation studies, to obtaining the views of people with dementia directly. There is now growing understanding from broader research in dementia care about the skills and techniques that can be used to give people with dementia opportunities to make their voices heard. Techniques that have been described in detail include: face-to-face interviews (Pratt 2002); telephone interviews (Mason and Wilkinson 2002); focus groups (Bamford and Bruce 2002); and video observation (Cook 2002).

There have also been suggestions (Cheston *et al.* 2000) that for people who cannot express their views directly, advocacy could have a role. The role of independent advocates in representing the views and interests of people with dementia would be different from that of proxies, who are generally not independent and whose perceptions of the person with dementia's views are more likely to be influenced by their own roles and interests.

Calls for more collaborative approaches to research with people with dementia (for example, Fryer 1999) have highlighted the politics of research in dementia care. Typically people with dementia and their families, as compared with professionals, researchers and research commissioners, have had little power or influence over the processes, outcomes or uses of research. One factor which might contribute to the redressing of this disempowerment is the growing pressure on researchers in the field of dementia care to apply the tenets of user involvement in research more generally.

Hanley *et al.* (2000) suggest a continuum encompassing three main ways in which people with dementia and their supporters might be involved in evaluations: consultation, collaboration and user control. For example, in the different approaches service users variously could be asked for their views about a proposed service evaluation; they might be invited to work alongside the evaluators to design, implement or act on the results of an evaluation; or they might undertake the evaluation with input from professional evaluators as and when they decide it is needed. Different types of involvement will be appropriate in different contexts; there is no one 'right' approach.

The most common form of user involvement in evaluative studies of dementia services, as with many other forms of research, is probably the inclusion of carers in the membership of the steering or advisory groups that are very often part of the evaluative process. The involvement of people with dementia in such groups is less frequent but is becoming more common. Such involvement needs to be planned and implemented carefully if people with dementia, and indeed carers, are to be enabled to participate fully. Much can be learned from more general guidance on involving service users in research (see, for example, Hanley *et al.* 2000) as well as from guidance on involving people with dementia in service development (Allan 2001; Cantley, Woodhouse and Smith 2005). In addition, evaluators in dementia care can learn from some innovative approaches to involving people with dementia in more broadly defined research. For example, Corner (2002) describes the practical operation and benefits of a user panel established to enable people with dementia to inform a study that aimed to develop a 'toolkit' of quality of life measures. This type of user panel approach could potentially be adapted for use in evaluative studies. However, Corner comments that this type of approach is resource intensive. This is an important consideration and will need to be addressed by those involved in designing and commissioning evaluations.

One of the interesting questions is whether we can expect to see user-controlled evaluation in dementia care. For carers, one of the main constraints in engaging in this way is likely to be the difficulty many will experience in taking time out from their caring role. The emergence of groups of people with dementia acting for and by themselves (for example, Dementia Advocacy and Support Network International and the Scottish

Dementia Working Group)[2] may bring nearer the prospect of user-controlled evaluation should such groups decide that engaging in service evaluation is a good way for them to influence the policy process.

Handling practical issues

There are numerous generic guides to the practical aspects of applying the range of research methods likely to be used by dementia care evaluators (for example, Clarke with Dawson 1999; Hall and Hall 2004; Patton 2002). However, from my experience of a range of dementia care evaluations there are also some practical problems that are particularly, but by no means exclusively, related to dementia care.

First, communication with people with dementia often takes more time as compared with other research participants. Evaluators need to ensure that sufficient time is built into studies and commissioners need to be prepared to provide the additional research time and resources.

Second, communications with people with dementia need to be tailored to their individual abilities and circumstances. There is evidence that even people with advanced dementia can communicate meaningfully if given the right opportunities (for example, Allan 2001; Hubbard *et al.* 2002; Killick and Allan 2001). However, one of the challenges for evaluators can be finding out enough about individuals in advance to accommodate their communication needs.

Third, there are often practical difficulties in gaining access to people with dementia and sometimes to carers. Carers, because of the very nature of their role, often find it difficult to find time, and substitute providers of care, to enable their participation. Carers and service providers are often, for the best of motives, protective and reluctant to allow the person with dementia time alone with researchers. Evaluators therefore need to build in time to work with such 'gatekeepers' to reassure them.

Fourth, one of the challenges for evaluators lies in ensuring that their studies take into account the diversity that exists amongst the population

---

2   For further information about these groups see the following websites: www.dasninternational.org and www.alzscot.org/pages/sdwg.htm.

of people with dementia relating to gender, age, sexuality, ethnicity, social and cultural backgrounds, and ability to express views about services. It should not be assumed that what works for some people with dementia will work for all. Evaluators need to consider two main areas. There is the evaluation of mainstream dementia services, where it is important that evaluators remember that there may be 'marginalized groups' of people with dementia whose perspective may be neglected (Innes, Archibald and Murphy 2004). For example, in an evaluation of a dementia day care service it might be important to take account of the perspectives of people within the local minority ethnic community, or those of younger people with dementia. Then there is the evaluation of specialist services set up to cater for marginalized groups. It is important to evaluate these specialist services and to take account in the conduct and use of these evaluations of similarities as well as differences from mainstream services. Without such comparison there is the risk that evaluations will serve to emphasize the ways in which minority groups are different and to under-state their similarities with users of mainstream services, so serving to reinforce their peripheral status (see Bowes and Wilkinson 2002). Ensuring the appropriate inclusion of marginalized groups in evaluations is likely to present additional challenges including, for example, examining issues of low take-up of services and gaining access to people who are not in contact with services, overcoming issues of language and cultural differences, and overcoming issues related to stigma.

Fifth, much dementia care is provided in settings which are small scale and often private, including domestic environments or 'private' locations in care homes, for example bedrooms and bathrooms. There is a considerable practical challenge for evaluators in assessing what goes on in these contexts while avoiding invasion of privacy or their presence affecting the course of events.

Sixth, evaluators need to consider many practical details in order to enable the full participation of people with dementia. For example, McKillop and Wilkinson (2004) provide advice from the perspective of people with dementia on issues including:

- ways to ensure the comfort of the person

- ways of ensuring a respectful and reciprocal relationship
- practical steps to make it easy for the person
- ways to 'make a graceful exit'.

Seventh, timing evaluations, particularly of innovative services, often poses problems. Such is the requirement for many new services to prove their worth, especially to those funding the services, that evaluation has become a routine requirement, often commissioned in the early stages of the service or even prior to its establishment. Evaluators need to consider carefully the appropriate timing for their work as if undertaken too early (a) they end up studying the process of setting up the service rather than its fully established operation and (b) the nature of the service may be evolving and the criteria for evaluation unclear.

Eighth, there can be practical difficulties associated with the demands of data gathering for staff when, as is often the case in dementia care, service resources are very stretched.

Ninth, the operation of dementia services is very often closely intertwined with the operation of other services in a broader service system. Typically such systems vary substantially from one locality to another. These factors mean that a wide range of service stakeholders may need to be involved in any evaluation, that it can be difficult to evaluate one service in isolation, and that it can be difficult to generalize findings from one locality to another.

Tenth, and finally, there are difficulties with terminology, particularly in the use of the words 'dementia' and 'carer'. Thus, not all relatives or other supporters of people with dementia consider themselves, or want others to consider them to be, a 'carer'. This is most evident in relation to relatives of people with early dementia. Similarly, some people with diagnoses, or their relatives, may object to use of the term 'dementia' or feel uncomfortable with it. Some people using identification, diagnosis and early support services may not know that dementia is a potential diagnosis; some people may not have been told, or may have forgotten the diagnosis; and some people using services that set out to 'normalize' people's experiences may not use the term. It can require great sensitivity on the part of the evaluator to ensure that the terminology used is appropriate.

Working ethically

Over the past decade or so the ethical approval of research in health and social care has assumed considerable prominence and the bureaucratic processes for the ethical approval of research have become commensurately more complicated.[3] Øvretveit (1998) suggests:

> The practical aims and the practice context in which evaluation is carried out create a greater potential for harm and conflict than many other types of research, and evaluation ethics are correspondingly more important. (p.195)

Much evaluation in dementia care involves respondents who are users or staff of NHS services. These evaluation studies must meet the ethical requirements for health services research. Health services research ethics procedures are shaped by assumptions about ethical issues and practices that are predominantly positivist and concerned with experimental and quantitative studies. This can make it difficult for evaluators using other methodologies to gain approval for their work and to access ethical advice that is appropriate to their activities. The development of separate research ethics procedures for social care research[4] may ease some of these problems.

The need for respondents to give informed consent to participation is one of the core requirements of ethical practice in health and social care evaluation. Again, for evaluators of dementia care there can be difficulties because of the dominance of the biomedical model, which gives rise to notions of competence and consent regarded as unduly narrow and restrictive from other perspectives on dementia. For example, in England the implementation of the Mental Capacity Act 2005 has implications for practice.

Alternative approaches to obtaining the consent of people with dementia have been developing. For example, Hubbard, Downs and

---

3   For further information see the Central Office for Research Ethics website: www.corec. org.uk.

4   Again, for further information see the Central Office for Research Ethics website: www.corec.org.uk.

Tester 2002) describe the processes they used for handling consent in relation to assessment of ability to consent and subsequently involving people who variously were deemed able or unable to give consent. They advocate that consent gathering be conceived as a continuous process rather than as a one-off event prior to participation. For other good practical descriptions of consent procedures see Allan (2001) and Dewing (2002).

McKillop and Wilkinson (2004) provide some practical advice from the perspective of a person with dementia regarding consent. Central to this advice is the need to make decisions based on individual circumstances, to respect the person with dementia's right to exercise choice about participation while being sensitive to the views of carers and avoiding creating difficulties.

Other ethical issues specifically relating to working with people with dementia include managing (see Stalker *et al.* 1999):

- the risk of unwanted intrusion into the lives of people with dementia

- the risk of generating emotional or other issues for individuals as a result of the processes of data collection raising their awareness or changing their thinking

- the risk of raising expectations of continuing friendships that will not be realized

- the pace and nature of withdrawal from people's lives

- confidentiality, especially where an individual appears to be at risk of harm

- the responsibility to put the information gathered to good use

- the need to give people something in return.

It is important to remember that these issues can apply equally to relatives and other supporters of those with dementia and many also apply to service providers who participate in evaluations. Bartlett and Martin (2002) provide a useful overview of ethical issues and ethical guidance in dementia care research.

In addition, from my own experience of undertaking a number of evaluation studies in dementia care, the following broader ethical difficulties are not uncommon:

- Managing to ensure that the findings of the evaluation are made available to all who contributed.

- Managing confidentiality and preservation of anonymity for service providers. This is particularly important when individuals or groups make critical comments about practice or about management in their own or other services.

- Managing criticisms of practice produced by the evaluation to try to ensure that they are not interpreted over-simplistically in allocating 'blame', a particular risk in relation to care staff who have limited training, status and power.

- Managing sensitively, but without compromise to the integrity of the evaluation, the way in which the commissioners and providers of innovative dementia care often have very considerable investments (ideological, professional, emotional, career, financial, organizational) in the evaluation producing positive findings and enter into the process wanting proof of worth rather than with openness to learning.

- Managing criticisms produced by the evaluation to try to ensure that they do not adversely affect morale and the drive to improve and innovate unduly. This is particularly an issue in dementia care because of the traditionally low status of services and low investment in service innovation and development.

Many of the ethical issues above arise from the ways in which the politics of evaluation generally (see Øvretveit 1998) are played out in the particular socio-political context of dementia care.

Conclusion

Bond and Corner (2001, p.97) argue 'that there are no unique methodological challenges in researching dementia or dementia care', and that:

…rather the complex nature of dementia and dementia care highlight the challenges we have in the investigation of any complex social phenomenon… Rather than the study of dementia and dementia care being difficult to study, it is the weakness of dominant methodological approaches and lack of theoretical rigour in health services research which militates against successful understanding and explanation of the phenomenon. (p.114)

My arguments in this chapter about evaluation have been broadly sympathetic to this view. While evaluating dementia care may not present unique methodological difficulties, it does pointedly illustrate difficulties and debates in the field of evaluation more generally. It also throws into sharp relief a specific range of technical, practical, political and ethical issues.

Certainly theoretical and methodological rigour is essential. But great care, and considerable sensitivity and skill, are also required to ensure that lessons learned in the broad field of evaluation research are tailored to the particular circumstances and requirements of dementia care. For, as I noted at the start of this chapter, the current political, economic and social policy contexts of dementia care lie at the root of the specific range of problems that affects this field of evaluation.

Acknowledgement

I am very grateful to Gilbert Smith for commenting on a draft of this chapter.

References

Aggarwal, N., Vass, A.A., Minardi, H.A., Ward, R., Garfield, C. and Cybyk, B. (2003) 'People with dementia and their relatives: personal experiences of Alzheimer's and the provision of care.' *Journal of Psychiatric and Mental Health Nursing 10*, 187–197.

Allan, K. (2001) *Communication and Consultation: Exploring Ways for Staff to Involve People with Dementia in Developing Services.* Bristol: Joseph Rowntree Foundation.

Bamford, C. and Bruce, E. (2000) 'Defining the outcomes of community care: the perspectives of older people with dementia and their carers.' *Ageing and Society 20*, 5, 543–570.

Bamford, C. and Bruce, E. (2002) 'Successes and challenges in using focus groups with older people with dementia.' In H. Wilkinson (ed.) *The Perspectives of People with Dementia: Research Methods and Motivations.* London: Jessica Kingsley Publishers.

Bartlett, H. and Martin, W. (2002) 'Ethical issues in dementia care research.' In H. Wilkinson (ed.) *The Perspectives of People with Dementia: Research Methods and Motivations.* London: Jessica Kingsley Publishers.

Bond, J. and Corner, L. (2001) 'Researching dementia: are there unique methodological challenges for health services research?' *Ageing and Society 21,* 1, 95–116.

Bond, J. and Corner, L. (2004) *Quality of Life and Older People.* Maidenhead: Open University Press.

Bowes, A. and Wilkinson, H. (2002) 'South Asian people with dementia.' In H. Wilkinson (ed.) *The Perspectives of People with Dementia: Research Methods and Motivations.* London: Jessica Kingsley Publishers.

Brooker, D. (2005) 'Dementia Care Mapping: a review of the literature.' *The Gerontologist 45,* Special Issue No. 1, 11–18.

Cantley, C., Woodhouse, J. and Smith, M. (2005) *Listen to Us: Involving People with Dementia in Service Planning and Development.* Newcastle upon Tyne: Dementia North, Northumbria University. Full text available from www.dementianorth.org.uk.

Challis, D., von Abendorff, R., Brown, P. and Chesterman, J. (1997) 'Care management and dementia: an evaluation of the Lewisham intensive case management scheme.' In S. Hunter (ed.) *Dementia: Challenges and New Directions.* London: Jessica Kingsley Publishers.

Cheston, R., Bender, M. and Byatt, S. (2000) 'Involving people who have dementia in the evaluation of services: a review.' *Journal of Mental Health 9,* 5, 471–479.

Chung, J.C.C. and Lai, C.K.Y. (2005) 'Snoezelen for dementia.' In *The Cochrane Database of Systematic Reviews, Issue 2.* Cochrane review abstract and plain language summary. www.cochrane.org/reviews/en/ab003152.html.

Clare, L., Woods, R.T., Moniz Cook, E.D., Orrell, M. and Spector, A. (2005) 'Cognitive rehabilitation and cognitive training for early-stage Alzheimer's disease and vascular dementia.' In *The Cochrane Database of Systematic Reviews, Issue 2.* Cochrane review abstract and plain language summary. www.cochrane.org/reviews/en/ab003260.html.

Clarke, A. with Dawson, R. (1999) *Evaluation Research: An Introduction to Principles, Methods and Practice.* London: Sage.

Cook, A. (2002) 'Using video observation to include the experiences of people with dementia in research.' In H. Wilkinson (ed.) *The Perspectives of People with Dementia: Research Methods and Motivations.* London: Jessica Kingsley Publishers.

Corner, L. (2002) 'Including people with dementia: advisory networks and user panels.' In H. Wilkinson (ed.) *The Perspectives of People with Dementia: Research Methods and Motivations.* London: Jessica Kingsley Publishers.

Dening, T. and Lawton, C. (1998) 'The role of carers in evaluating mental health services for older people.' *International Journal of Geriatric Psychiatry 13,* 863–870.

Dewing, J. (2002) 'From ritual to relationship: a person-centred approach to consent in qualitative research with older people who have a dementia.' *Dementia 1,* 2, 157–171.

Downs, M. (1997) 'Evaluating dementia services.' In M. Marshall (ed.) *State of the Art in Dementia Care.* London: Centre for Policy on Ageing.

Everitt, A. and Hardiker, P. (1996) *Evaluating for Good Practice.* Basingstoke and London: Macmillan.

Forbes, D., Morgan, D.G., Bangma, J., Peacock, S., Pelletier, N. and Adamson, J. (2005) 'Light therapy for managing sleep, behaviour, and mood disturbances in dementia.'

In *The Cochrane Database of Systematic Reviews, Issue 2.* Cochrane review abstract and plain language summary. www.cochrane.org/reviews/en/ab003946.html.

Fryer, D. (1999) 'Commentary.' In K. Stalker, J. Gilliard and M. Downs 'Eliciting user perspectives on what works.' *International Journal of Geriatric Psychiatry 14*, 120–134.

Gilliard, J. (2001) 'The perspectives of people with dementia, their families and carers.' In C. Cantley (ed.) *A Handbook of Dementia Care.* Buckingham: Open University Press.

Guba, E.G. and Lincoln, Y.S. (1989) *Fourth Generation Evaluation.* Newbury Park, California: Sage.

Hall, I. and Hall, D. (2004) *Evaluation and Social Research: Introducing Small-Scale Practice.* Basingstoke: Palgrave Macmillan.

Hancock, G.A., Reynolds, T., Woods, B., Thornicroft, G. and Orrell, M. (2003) 'The needs of older people with mental health problems according to the user, carer and the staff.' *International Journal of Geriatric Psychiatry 18*, 803–811.

Hanley, B., Bradburn, J., Gorin, S., Barnes, M., Evans, C., Goodare, H., Kelson, M., Kent, A., Oliver, S. and Wallcraft, J. (2000) *Involving Consumers in Research and Development in the NHS: Briefing Notes for Researchers.* Winchester: Consumers in the NHS Research Support Unit, The Help for Health Trust.

Hubbard, G., Cook, A., Tester, S. and Downs, M. (2002) 'Beyond words: older people with dementia using and interpreting nonverbal behaviour.' *Journal of Ageing Studies 16*, 2, 155–167.

Hubbard, G., Downs, M. and Tester, S. (2002) 'Including the perspectives of older people in institutional care during the consent process.' In H. Wilkinson (ed.) *The Perspectives of People with Dementia: Research Methods and Motivations.* London: Jessica Kingsley Publishers.

Innes, A., Archibald, C. and Murphy, C. (eds) (2004) *Dementia and Social Inclusion: Marginalised Groups and Marginalised Areas of Dementia Research, Care and Practice.* London: Jessica Kingsley Publishers.

Killick, J. and Allan, K. (2001) *Communication and the Care of People with Dementia.* Buckingham: Open University Press.

Kitwood, T. (1997) *Dementia Reconsidered: The Person Comes First.* Buckingham: Open University Press.

Levin, E., Sinclair, I. and Gorbach, P. (1983) *The Supporters of Confused Elderly Persons at Home: Extract for the Main Report.* London: National Institute for Social Work Research Unit.

Loveman, E., Green, C., Kirby, J., Takeda, A., Picot, J., Payne, E. and Clegg, A. (2004) *The Clinical and Cost-effectiveness of Donepezil, Rivastigmine, Galantamine, Memantine for Alzheimer's Disease: Technology Assessment Report Commissioned by the HTA Programme on behalf of The National Institute for Clinical Excellence.* Southampton: Southampton Health Technology Assessments Centre.

Mason, A. and Wilkinson, H. (2002) 'Don't leave me hanging on the telephone: interviews with people with dementia using the telephone.' In H. Wilkinson (ed.) *The Perspectives of People with Dementia: Research Methods and Motivations.* London: Jessica Kingsley Publishers.

McKillop, J. and Wilkinson, H. (2004) 'Make it easy on yourself! Advice to researchers from someone with dementia on being interviewed.' *Dementia 3*, 2, 117–125.

Moriarty, J. and Webb, S. (2000) *Part of their Lives: Community Care for Older People with Dementia.* Bristol: The Policy Press.

Murphy, E., Dingwall, R., Greatbatch, D., Parker, S. and Watson, P. (1998) 'Qualitative research methods in health technology assessment: a review of the literature.' *Health Technology Assessment 2,* 16, 1–274.

National Institute for Clinical Excellence (NICE) (2001) *Guidance on the Use of Donepezil, Rivastigmine and Galantamine for the Treatment of Alzheimer's Disease:Technology Appraisal Guidance – No.19.* London: National Institute for Clinical Excellence. www.nice.org. uk/page.aspx?o=14400.

National Institute for Health and Clinical Excellence (NIHCE) (2005) Extracts from the unpublished *Final Appraisal Determination in the appraisal of Donepezil, Rivastigmine, Galantamine and Memantine for the treatment of Alzheimer's Disease.* www.nice.org.uk/page.aspx?o=268171.

Neal, M. and Briggs, M. (2005) 'Validation therapy for dementia.' In *The Cochrane Database of Systematic Reviews, Issue 2.* Cochrane review abstract and plain language summary. www.cochrane.org/reviews/en/ab001394.html.

Nocon, A. and Qureshi, H. (1996) *Outcomes of Community Care for Users and Carers: A Social Services Perspective.* Buckingham: Open University Press.

Novella, J.L., Jochum, C., Jolly, D., Morrone, I., Ankin, J., Bureau, F. and Blanchard, F. (2001) 'Agreement between patients' and proxies' reports of quality of life in Alzheimer's disease.' *Quality of Life Research 10,* 5, 443–452.

Øvretveit, J. (1998) *Evaluating Health Interventions.* Buckingham: Open University Press.

Parlett, M. and Hamilton, D. (1977) 'Evaluation as illumination: a new approach to the study of innovatory programmes.' In D. Hamilton, D. Jenkins, C. King, B. MacDonald and M. Parlett (eds) *Beyond the Numbers Game: A Reader in Educational Evaluation.* Basingstoke: Macmillan.

Patton, M.Q. (2002) *Qualitative Research and Evaluation Methods* (Third edition). London: Sage.

Pawson, R. and Tilley, N. (1997) *Realistic Evaluation.* London: Sage.

Pratt, R. (2002) 'Nobody's ever asked me how I felt.' In H. Wilkinson (ed.) *The Perspectives of People with Dementia: Research Methods and Motivations.* London: Jessica Kingsley Publishers.

Pritchard, E.J. and Dewing, J. (2001) 'A multi-method evaluation of an independent dementia care service and its approach.' *Aging and Mental Health 5,* 1, 63–72.

Richards, K., Moniz-Cook, E., Duggan, P., Carr, I. and Wang, M. (2003) 'Defining "early dementia" and monitoring intervention: what measures are useful in family caregiving?' *Aging and Mental Health 7,* 1, 7–14.

Smith, G. and Cantley, C. (1985) *Assessing Health Care: A Study in Organizational Evaluation.* Buckingham: Open University Press.

Smith, S.C., Lampling, D.L., Banerjee, S., Harwood, R., Foley, B., Smith, P., Cook, J.C., Murray, J., Prince, M., Levin, E., Mann, A. and Knapp, M. (2005a) 'Measurement of health-related quality of life for people with dementia: development of a new instrument (DEMQOL) and an evaluation of current methodology.' *Health Technology Assessment 9,* 10.

Smith, S.C., Murray, J., Banerjee, S., Foley, B., Cook, J.C., Lamping, D.L., Prince, M., Harwood, R.H., Levin, E. and Mann, A. (2005b) 'What constitutes health-related quality of life in dementia? Development of a conceptual framework for people with dementia and their carers.' *International Journal of Geriatric Psychiatry 20*, 889–895.

Spencer, L., Ritchie, J., Lewis, J. and Dillon, L. (2003) *Quality in Qualitative Evaluation: A Framework for Assessing Research Evidence.* London: Government Chief Social Researcher's Office.

Stalker, K., Gilliard, J. and Downs, M. (1999) 'Eliciting user perspectives on what works.' *International Journal of Geriatric Psychiatry 14*, 120–134.

Thompson, L. (2005) 'Is it possible to conceptualise and measure quality of life for people with severe Alzheimer's Disease?' *Generations Review 15*, 1, 22–24.

Thorgrimsen, L., Spector, A., Wiles, A. and Orrell, M. (2005) 'Aroma therapy for dementia.' In *The Cochrane Database of Systematic Reviews, Issue 2.* Cochrane review abstract and plain language summary. www.cochrane.org/reviews/en/ab003150.html.

Traynor, V., Pritchard, E. and Dewing, J. (2004) 'Illustrating the importance of including the views and experiences of users and carers in evaluating the effectiveness of drug treatments for dementia.' *Dementia 3*, 2, 145–159.

Vink, A.C., Birks, J.S., Bruinsma, M.S. and Scholten, R.J.S. (2005) 'Music therapy for people with dementia.' In *The Cochrane Database of Systematic Reviews, Issue 2.* Cochrane review abstract and plain language summary. www.cochrane.org/reviews/en/ab003477.html.

Woods, B., Spector, A., Jones, C., Orrell, M. and Davies, S. (2005) 'Reminiscence therapy for dementia.' In *The Cochrane Database of Systematic Reviews, Issue 2.* Cochrane review abstract and plain language summary. www.cochrane.org/reviews/en/ab001120.html.

Chapter 3

Internal versus External Evaluation

Carolyn Lechner

When dementia care providers elect to evaluate the quality of the care they offer, one aspect they must consider is who will best evaluate the setting – insiders or external personnel? The selection could potentially be contingent on other subjective understandings – such as who the stakeholders are when the situation centres around the delivery of long-term dementia care. Evaluation has become popular to ascertain the quality of life and/or care of people with dementia. As observation tools such as Dementia Care Mapping (Bradford Dementia Group 1997) and the Alzheimer's Disease-Related Quality of Life instrument (ADRQL) (Black, Rabins and Kasper 2000; Rabins, Lyketsos and Steel 1999) have evolved in their appeal and application in certain settings that were previously difficult to measure, aspects such as the effectiveness of the evaluator have garnered more consideration. Whether the evaluation is internal or external may have a great deal to do with whether the impetus for change is also internal or external. This choice seems to speak to the culture of the organization.

The provision of care for people with dementia has entered an era of change. Advocates in the realm of dementia and nursing home care are joining forces around the world to bring about change in the fundamental ways long-term care is delivered and perceived. With this shifting concept of care, new questions emerge regarding how to conduct an evaluation. How to include the views of the person with dementia? Who is the evaluation for? What will the outcomes of evaluation be? The manner in which an evaluation is conducted sends a message regarding expectations of care in the future.

Definition of stakeholders

The selection of whether an external or internal evaluation will best meet the needs of the evaluation largely depends upon whom the facility considers to be the stakeholders in the dementia care setting. One report suggests that stakeholders are those who provide the service and those who use it (Walker *et al.* 2001). Stakeholders are those who have an interest in the outcome of an evaluation. Certain representatives of the modern age of culture change suggest that stakeholders are: people with dementia, families, advocates, staff and surveyors (Lustbader 2001). Surely there will be different stakeholders served by the same project who nonetheless have different goals. Despite these discrepancies, ultimately stakeholders must agree on the criteria of programme success.

Posavac and Carey (1992) stress the importance of comprehensive planning prior to the commencement of an evaluation, in order to get the outcome most directly related to one's setting. Step one in their six-step process of planning an evaluation is to identify stakeholders. They also suggest that there can be stakeholders who cannot participate in the same manner as their peers but their claim is no less valid.

In their consideration of programme evaluation, sociologists Rossi and Freeman (1993) discuss the 'social ecology of evaluations' and consider that participating in an evaluation is a fragile process fraught with numerous pitfalls – first, recognizing that all stakeholders do not speak the same language. Questions must be asked: Who are the disenfranchised? Staff have not always been considered worthy of holding a claim as stakeholder. What are the barriers to participation in the evaluation? Are they physical, such as for those investors who have a stake but are not present in the facility to monitor the evaluation, and social? For if a class strata still exists in which staff voices are perceived as less significant, then hurdles do indeed exist. Whose perspective should evaluators take? Are recipients of care able to make their voices heard? Is there any conflict among stakeholders?

In addition to stakeholders, Stake (2004) notes that there is also the concept of an audience, or those who will pay attention to the evaluator's findings. A staff member whose work in the dementia care setting is evaluated can find themselves to be both. Consequently, one staff member receiving feedback acts as both audience member and stakeholder: as a member of the audience hearing recommendations for the first time, a great deal of enthusiasm could be generated about the picture that is being presented. On the other hand, the stakeholder side of the staff member may be inclined to be more cynical and will not be swayed by the vision if significant change is demanded. Stakeholders have thanked me for feedback I have offered, stating that the plan for improvement is an encouraging ideal to strive for but is in no way realistic and that they will just keep doing what they have been doing. One corporate care provider wistfully told me after a very preliminary, initial presentation of what an evaluation could ultimately do for their organization that they were so far away from what I proposed that they could never see how to realistically get from 'point A to point B' and so terminated our contract at that time.

Is the culture of long-term care ready for the potential upheaval that evaluation feedback could create? In informal terms, are they ready to 'walk the walk'? It is imperative the evaluators consider that recommendations need to be kept within the psychological reach of the stakeholders. Cases have emerged when the changes proposed are so profound that administrators and staff have abandoned the evaluation process altogether in discouragement. Posavac and Carey (1992) stress that 'evaluation is best carried out when evaluators and stakeholders are explicit about their values and examine the effect of value presuppositions on evaluation procedures and interpretations' (p.255).

External evaluation

Assets

The duty of external evaluators appears linear and singular in its purpose: their own task is to find out if, how and why the programme is working. In dementia-specific and other long-term care programmes, the degree of effectiveness is no longer utilized solely as a marketing tool in which word of mouth spreads and beds are filled, but rather considered a mandate at state and national levels (see Chapter 4 for further discussion). Consultants who have been trained to identify which programmes meet certain key criteria can do so quickly. These individuals are not constrained by reporting findings to a programme manager who acts as supervisor. Subsequently, no reason exists for the evaluator to feel obligated to alter their data to reflect more favourable results (Krause 1996).

The difference between internal and external evaluations can even be determined on a theoretical level. Certain scholars (Rossi and Freeman 1993; Stake 2004) delineate the difference between a summative and formative evaluation process. The former is used when administrative decision makers are looking to specifically measure the presence or absence of certain aspects of a given programme. For this reason, in dementia care, a most likely form of summative evaluation would be at the level of the survey conducted by the local or regulatory governing board.

It is probable, however, that most instances of dementia care evaluation would instead fall under the category of formative evaluation, or an evaluation which plans to strengthen the strategy for service delivery, to raise the outcomes of programmes, or to increase the efficiency of services (Posavac and Carey 1992). The fundamental focus of this approach is to assess the competence of staff to carry out certain daily tasks on behalf of their residents in a manner which affirms their personhood.

Rossi and Freeman (1993) suggest that evaluations conducted today would not have been so readily offered to facility staff in recent decades: the 'old culture' (Kitwood 1997) of dementia care presumed that hired staff could not possess personal insights about how to attain well-being for both the residents and the facility. While this has changed for the most part, there are regrettably still facilities who hold this philosophy. Those researchers concerned about the integrity, validity and respectability of the results may believe that using externally selected evaluators is the best solution to the problem.

Rossi and Freeman (1993) suggest that accountability may be an issue when a facility ponders the selection of an internal or external evaluation. The two formats are generally aligned with different research methodologies: quantitative methods complement external evaluation styles, while internal evaluations are offered richness via qualitative methods. Researchers in dementia care who are still sceptical of the validity of qualitative findings appear to favour strongly the external evaluation format. Doyle (1992) argues, 'Independent evaluations are the only way that properly designed, scientifically valid studies can take place' (p.15).

In 2005, the US Alzheimer's Association initiated a national campaign whose goal is to build 'consensus among care experts, industry and professional groups, and Association chapters'. Through the use of various evidence-based projects currently underway (www.alz.org) the outcome will be practice recommendations in two areas: that of the best method to promote advocacy and public policy; and that of the best means of delivering optimal processes for training and self-evaluation. Since the Association is itself an agency external to the long-term care model of dementia care, an external evaluation becomes a logical mode of collecting information.

At this time in the territory of dementia care, several instruments are emerging which attempt to capture the essence of the dementia care setting. Many of these are administered by trained study research assistants and care professionals, and will involve the use of clinical staff, but as proxies for conveying resident conditions only, not as research collectors. For example, in a special edition of *The Gerontologist* published in 2005, Sloane, Zimmerman and other researchers who have devoted time to improving dementia care gathered together to consider the state of modern dementia care. They write 'being able to capture a clearer image of quality of life throughout the illness will help guide treatment and, ultimately, improve the experience of persons with the disease, their families, and those who provide their care' (Sloane *et al.* 2005, p.39). As this work is heavily focused on treatment, it can greatly enhance those evaluative tools which seek to understand more about the fundamental exchanges which take place during daily care interactions between all participants in the dementia care setting, people with dementia and staff alike.

In this same issue, Edelman *et al.* (2005) examined a variety of dementia-specific tools (see Table 3.1) to assess their effectiveness in measuring quality of life in dementia care settings. Some of these measures

Table 3.1 Dementia-specific quality of life measurement instruments

The Resident Quality of Life – Alzheimer's Disease instrument (Resident QOL-AD) (Logsdon et al. 2000)

- 13-item structured interview
- meant to assess relationships, physical condition and mood
- tested on individuals with dementia still residing in the community as well as their families

The Staff QOL-AD Quality of Life – Alzheimer's Disease instrument (Staff QOL-AD) (Logsdon et al. 2000)

- this is the staff proxy companion to the Resident QOL-AD

The Alzheimer's Disease-Related Quality of Life instrument (ADRQL) (Black et al. 2000; Rabins et al. 1999)

The Dementia Quality of Life instrument (DQoL) (Brod et al. 1999)

- 30-item interview consisting of five subscales

Dementia Care Mapping (DCM) (Bradford Dementia Group 1997)

- involves observing people with dementia at five-minute intervals and coding them in regard to their behaviours and levels of well-being

---

were administered to direct care providers, but specifically as a correlate to the relationship that a provider has with individuals with dementia.

In recent years, private, for-profit research groups with social programmes as their primary focus have emerged to meet the needs of dementia care facilities who are eagerly seeking new ways to change the manner in which care is provided. As concern has increased about the quality of life for people with dementia, external experts have become desirable to facilities in great need of a fundamental shift in culture.

(The potential advantages of external evaluators are summarized in Table 3.2.)

Drawbacks

The most basic problem the external evaluator faces when entering a dementia-specific setting to complete an evaluation are perceptions among individuals with dementia and staff alike that 'outsiders' or 'strangers' are present on the floor. This foreign, if benign, presence will almost certainly have some impact on the behaviour of staff and residents alike. Whether the change is significant enough to reflect a false impression of how care is provided in the setting has much to do with the rapport that the evaluator(s) are able to establish prior to the beginning of the evaluation.

While the insights of external evaluators may offer unique and important perspectives to staff during the feedback process, most facilities cannot or will not offer the resources necessary to allow external evaluators the opportunity to remain present at the site for any length of time beyond the completion of the feedback session with staff. I have had interaction with unit managers who openly admit that they are looking for a 'quick fix': their unit has been cited by a regulatory body, a complaint has been made by a family member, and they need to indicate that progress has been made. Yet, once these external agents have been appeased, these units probably revert to former practice, as they have no investment in a long-term change in culture.

As a result, it would be fairly difficult to forge any kind of supportive rapport between clinical staff and evaluative personnel which could get a useful dialogue started over time (Muller-Hergl 2003). A facility would have to have an unusual commitment to either change or research for them to invest in the kind of pre-test/post-test style of evaluative practice that would last for an extended time. Instead, what many facilities are faced with is a 'one-off' evaluation of care, where in ideal circumstances feedback can be shared with all staff. Most likely, though, this is a model scenario, as staff cannot always commit to compromising staffing ratios on the floor in order to be present with peers to hear the feedback in a team setting. Even if all staff are present, the evaluator(s) must then leave, and maintaining a commitment to a potentially better yet often more time-consuming plan of care is generally abandoned in favour of efficiency.

An external evaluator may be blind to certain implicit elements of a local culture which could inform results, and, without insights in to local customs and slang, could be interpreting interactions incorrectly. Also an external evaluator may have expectations about access that are not in keeping with the organization, which may have an interest in discretion.

For example, a dementia care setting may negotiate somewhat non-traditional plans of care with a resident that are not in keeping with local regulations, but which bring greater levels of well-being to an individual with dementia. External evaluators may not see the value in such an exchange (for example, a resident who elects not to shave every day, but who agrees to shave every third day, could be a conflict for regulations related to hygiene, but if intentions are stated clearly in care plans, this may cease to be an issue).

Furthermore, an external evaluator may misinterpret specific elements which, for whatever reason, are constructed by the agency because they work: the external evaluator may have a vision for the ideal which is not shared by the group they are studying (Stake 2004). For example, a facility where people with dementia can choose to remain in pyjamas well into the morning may be perceived as neglectful of its care of residents who should be dressed and clean by breakfast. Perhaps the facility has discovered that residents who are able to determine that they would like to dress on their own are much less combative and more comfortable than residents who are dressed and bathed at the discretion of staff with heavy workloads (Twigg 2000).

An external evaluation sometimes reveals the frequent, but important, discrepancies between the way that dementia programmes are formally described to the community, the way that dementia programmes are thought to operate by administrative staff and families, and how these programmes truly operate in reality. An organization where change is gradually gaining acceptance in which seeds of potential are being sown may not be prepared for the scrutiny and judgement which an external evaluation may yield (Rossi and Freeman 1993). Administrations who have seen glimpses of practice which reflect the new culture of care seek to participate in these customs themselves. But administrative staff cannot expect to ask staff to treat residents with person-centred care if they are not feeling cared for themselves (Baker, Edwards and Packer 2003a).

Also, external evaluators will lack the fluency in the 'language' of a facility which could truncate the amount of pertinent, care-related infor-mation which is worthy and able to be collected, reviewed and dissemi-nated to staff. Because of the highly transient nature of dementia care work, floor staff may express scepticism of 'outsiders' who arrive, collect data over a short time, and present a plan for change, regardless of how enthusiastic these individuals may be. There is a 'been there, done that' attitude that staff reserve for every new plan for care which is introduced as 'the solution', because so often these new ideas are themselves overhauled for new plans within a matter of months. I have found it to be extremely beneficial to do some informal research about the facility to whom I am providing feedback. Have there been some significant changes in the way care has been provided in the last several months? Specifically, what were those changes? Am I asking staff to consider a major shift in care provision which I think is new and innovative but which staff already tried and abandoned two years ago? Staff who remain in the setting for any amount of time may become cynical of all change, particularly when it lauds 'a new way of thinking' (Lawton 2001).

The potential disadvantages of external evaluators are summarized in Table 3.2.

Table 3.2 Potential advantages and disadvantages of external evaluators

Potential advantages of external evaluators
- evaluators are already trained so may be more efficient
- evaluators would feel less administrative pressure to report a certain way
- external evaluations are generally summative; the goal is to assess staff competence to complete daily tasks
- external evaluations may preserve the greatest degree of validity

Potential disadvantages of external evaluators
- external evaluators could elicit false performance from staff
- external evaluators may not understand unique unit culture
- external evaluators may not appreciate unit history

Internal evaluation

Ethics

An internal evaluation in a dementia setting demands that a certain degree of training must take place before staff can begin to ensure the safety and dignity of individuals with dementia in the evaluation process. Staff may wish to review their facility's philosophy of care in order to focus on what the intentions of the evaluations may be. Without this moral foundation, evaluation can develop into a dangerous entity.

Jennings (2000) discusses the ethical component and moral imperative of trying to deliver quality of life to people with dementia. If quality of life is considered to be a benchmark and concept of evaluation, the assessment is of the process, not the recipient of care. Krause (1996) likewise notes that the ethics of evaluation is as much about the prevention of exploitation of residents as it is about the character of those conducting research. In a 2001 'think tank' held in Bradford, UK, several advocates of the Dementia Care Mapping method discussed how the method could be potentially renamed 'care mapping' so it would more accurately focus on the subject of care provision rather than scrutiny of residents' behaviour as problematic (Brooker and Rogers 2001).

Stake (2004) suggests that the role of evaluator is infused with ethical issues which they must enthusiastically address. Are they conveying the most accurate picture of the setting with the least amount of tension added to the daily lives of people with dementia and staff? Furthermore, if role conflict exists on the part of the staff member-turned-evaluator, is the individual capable of determining appropriate allegiance in a satisfactory manner?

Finally, it is possible that administrators may deliberately select certain caregivers to be evaluators with the idea that these unique personalities could help them work through their scepticism. These individuals are selected for qualities leadership feels may help answer questions such as: Is change possible? Is our setting worthy of change and the effort which would accompany such conditions?

Assets

Several practical reasons exist which could explain why a facility would opt for the use of internal evaluators. Cost and time are just two key areas which would immediately be served by such a decision. Internal evaluators in dementia care settings would already have knowledge about many fundamental elements such as the layout of the facility, insights into how to avoid agitating residents and how best to support others. Hiring staff as evaluators would tend to be a more efficient choice, and there would be no need to orientate evaluators in an effort to catch up. Very likely, staff would be more thorough in less time, and with greater sensitivity (Krause 1996). Instead of familiarizing themselves with where things are located and of what the daily routine is comprised, staff can instead be spending that time asking themselves what they might hope for as an outcome of the evaluation – what are the areas that need work or greater consideration?

Internal evaluators face internal challenges at the outset of their work, in that they must be approved as trustworthy and insightful not only by leadership, but also by the staff team on the floor. Administrators have an advantage at this stage as well, because the staff they select to complete the evaluation are known entities – selected for their knowledge of every aspect of the programme, their compassion and their resourcefulness. Ultimately, these selected evaluators will usually find the programme directors and staff more open to constructive criticism which could emerge from the evaluation as well as potentially more willing to acknowledge areas which could benefit from improvement.

Internal evaluators have an advantage in the recommendations they offer to staff because they will be able to personally monitor the implementation of their ideas. Finally, in being selected, these staff-turned-evaluators will gain understanding that their contribution means something, and will then devote more time and attention to the project, as they realize they have become a true stakeholder in the setting (Posavac and Carey 1992).

In addition, some of those staff not selected may internalize this slight and could even manifest their frustration by denigrating this effort of their peers to others as ineffective and amateur and could even go so far as to sabotage the evaluator's efforts. On the other hand, staff who are not selected subsequently have daily contact with a staff member who has been given trust and responsibility by administration. Using these individuals as models for one's performance ensures organizational change at yet another level. To be sure, assuming the role of internal evaluator greatly increases one's sense of responsibility and accountability to one's community (Rossi and Freeman 1993).

If a facility desires to ensure that the care provided is meeting national guidelines, it is probable that the impartial judgement of an external evaluation is what is needed to ensure that quality of care is being delivered at satisfactory levels. For day-to-day care planning purposes, however, an internal evaluation may be more complementary to a dementia care setting than an external evaluation. The intention of an internal evaluation is more in keeping with currently evolving philosophies that suggest that problem-solving is most successful when originated from dementia care staff – it is suggested that this practice is successful because it becomes proactive: staff see how their own plans can feasibly prevent certain problems before they occur. The well-being of people with dementia shifts every day and is met in different ways every day. Insightful care can reflect this (Alzheimer's Association 2005).

Truly progressive facilities may elect to conduct an internal evaluation for the sole purpose of empowering staff to make their own decisions toward finding their own solutions. By encouraging staff to find new solutions, administration is giving the staff ownership of those solutions, giving them motivation to monitor their own care plans and to assess their effectiveness. Staff see their own imprint on the residents across the care process. When administrations determine that the best solutions can be found within, they send a message to their staff and infuse the resolution with greater power.

In 2002 and 2003, Baker, Edwards and Packer wrote a five-part series in *The Journal of Dementia Care* which focused on Dementia Care Mapping as a benchmarking tool. These authors explain that 'evaluating person-centered care requires us as caregivers to focus on the unique experience of care from a person's point of view' (Baker and Edwards 2002, p.23). Additionally, they state that through the process of evaluation, each staff member gets a greater overall understanding of his or her own role (Baker, Edwards and Packer 2003b). If Dementia Care Mapping (DCM) is selected as the specific method of internal evaluation, it may increase the legitimacy of this choice since its data are quantitative and many critics feel that statistical evidence is key (Walker *et al.* 2001). Additionally, with

DCM, there is a greater likelihood that evaluation will be used in conjunction with other elements such as feedback to staff and action planning for the future (Brooker 2002).

Since formative evaluations are conducted with the implicit understanding that they will produce plans for action, it follows reasonably that internal evaluation would be expressed in a manner which would be most logical to other staff, since it is understood that they speak the same language and share the same culture. Plans for improving care are generated internally, will make more sense, and will be able to be implemented sooner. Rossi and Freeman (1993) note that internal evaluation offers the staff member-turned-evaluator the chance to evolve further into the role of advocate for the individuals with dementia who reside in the setting.

In the same way that external for-profit agencies specifically constructed to offer evaluations have emerged for the facilities that need them, many facilities and service agencies that provide regular dementia care have created in-house staff positions in research to make periodic evaluations possible. Care must be taken when integrating these new research specialists with clinical staff, though, because without effort, even employees of the same organization can perceive each other as outsiders and unworthy of support.

(The potential advantages of internal evaluators are summarized in Table 3.3.)

Drawbacks

Despite certain facets which would greatly enhance dementia care, internal evaluations have their own detractions. Care must be taken in preparation to ascertain that internal evaluators do not fall victim to several potential pitfalls. One may question the integrity of an evaluator who receives payment from the very organization they are meant to evaluate (Krause 1996). A malevolent culture could convey a message of intimidation. Instead of assessing conditions in an environment fostering freedom and choice, these evaluators could potentially fall victim to internal pressure, ultimately conveying a message not of their own choosing but which perhaps portrays an image the administration finds favourable but in no way reflects the true condition of the environment.

Internal evaluations might also be compromised by confused evaluators with good intentions. Krause (1996) notes that it is because there is such an investment on the part of every caregiver that one might expect a certain degree of bias to infuse itself, however subconsciously, into the impressions of the internal staff evaluator. Should an evaluator come across a caregiving situation in which a caregiver performs in a significantly substandard manner, one so poor that the worker's ongoing employment is in question, the untrained evaluator may struggle with reporting the findings which will implicate this individual and perhaps lead to suspension or termination. Not only do these individuals potentially not want to make these decisions, they almost certainly do not want to be identified as the individual responsible for recording and reporting this information.

Reluctance on the part of an internal evaluator may stem less from an altruistic desire to protect one's co-workers and more from a self-preservation oriented drive. An insightful evaluator may discover during their course of study that certain harmful elements run through the setting which, if discovered, could potentially yield change at a level of concern to warrant a complete overhaul of staff structure. If their own professional livelihood is challenged, an internal evaluator may be hard pressed to reveal their findings without at least being tempted to 'sugar-coat' findings (Posavac and Carey 1992). I have found that the most effective way to present findings that are less than favourable in a feedback situation is diplomatically – condescension will eliminate any rapport one could establish. Rather, showing a willingness to hear the frustrations of staff is important.

The use of DCM as an evaluative method may create unpleasant dynamics for certain staff members if they are selected to be mappers, because traditional day-to-day dynamics would not demand that these individuals enter into the potentially confrontational interactions with fellow co-workers that the feedback segment of DCM can create. Because of the highly stressful nature of work in the dementia setting, caregivers often look to their peers for support. If the culture of the organization is not yet at a place where criticism can be made and taken constructively, then tension emerges. Some believe that many dementia facilities may discover DCM and eagerly initiate evaluation using it. Muller-Hergl (2003) argues that DCM is one observation tool which is yet too powerful for most settings. 'The professional care field is not prepared for the kind of learning that DCM demands. This results in useless feedback and initiates the slow death of the method' (Muller-Hergl 2003, p.65). Without comprehensive staff training and complete embrace of person-centred philosophy, the tool will only be successful among the long-term care élite.

Without comprehensive training, the rich feedback that results from a comprehensive DCM evaluation is only 'interesting' to staff who are receiving the recommendations. The changes often cannot be implemented in the setting because most staff do not feel that they have the power or time to initiate such profound change. Instead of fostering a greater sense of team, those staff who have been selected to be mappers can come across to staff as 'experts' who have entered a different plane of communication with administrative staff. If certain staff are already feeling overwhelmed by their work and that administration does not hear their needs or ideas, that attempts to change and improve care would be futile, this will only alienate them more (Muller-Hergl 2003).

Muller-Hergl (2003) also challenges the idea that an internal evaluation will save an organization the time and money that an external evaluation would demand. If an internal evaluation is as thorough as DCM, with the intentions of making changes at such a fundamental level that attitudes and philosophies must change, then truly more time would be taken instructing future mappers that they possess a tool with great power which must be used with great care (Brooker and Rogers 2001).

There are certain occasions where the nature of internal evaluation has little value. For the culture of long-term care truly to change, quality dementia care must be able to be disseminated across numerous settings. If evaluation is meant to implement standards of care across several homes, the personalized element of knowing the facility may lose some of its relevance (Baker, Edwards and Packer 2003a).

Some elements related to the drawbacks of an internal evaluation may have to do with over-confidence or a lack of insight into the complexities of changing an entire culture of care. An internal evaluator may feel that he has such an implicit understanding of the programme in question that he will overlook certain important fundamental features about the programme (Stake 2004). Conversely, staff involved in internal evaluation may have so little faith in those who chose them that they do not believe that their concerns will be heard. This is why, in order for internal evaluation to be effective, organizational change may be necessary (Walker *et al.* 2001).

I have found that greatest success has come when an organization embraces organizational change 'from the top down'. Themes in this chapter suggest that each care provider must embrace a core change in their understanding about how to enact change ('I am an agent of change') and that it would be fitting to see a second-shift carer approach a unit manager with a proposal for systemic change for the unit. In reality this has not proven to be the prevalent model for organizational change. I have, however, seen administrative level staff who 'walk the walk' of organizational change by distributing decision-making power to staff at all levels. These individuals seem to understand that change does not occur overnight, and that to improve care for residents, care for staff must be considered as well.

An additional dilemma of internal evaluations emerges when professional stakeholders express doubt regarding the authenticity of findings. For this reason, the most comprehensive programme evaluation could be one which is both internal and external (Rossi and Freeman 1993), one that uses internal evaluators but which employs consultants who can provide both technical assistance and an overview. In this framework, the site being evaluated gets the benefit of data which has been collected by local staff and possesses all of the insights they would have to offer, but which has also been screened and reviewed for its merit by experts.

Recognition of the many processes that comprise the evaluation process is critical – collection of data in a particular fashion and then determining that it does or does not meet certain criteria is merely the first step in a complex course of action. Criticism, if delivered in the right relation with the staff to whom it is directed, can be the first step toward exciting and positive change. Yet, staff selected to offer feedback may come into the exchange completely unprepared to offer feedback to staff eager to hear impressions of their day-to-day work (Brooker 2002).

The potential disadvantages of internal evaluators are summarized in Table 3.3.

Table 3.3 Potential advantages and disadvantages of internal evaluators

Potential advantages of internal evaluators
- evaluators' familiarity with setting could save time and money
- evaluators are a known entity, selected for their skills and insight
- evaluators can monitor implementation of any plan in the long term
- evaluators are examples of staff empowerment and potential for organizational change

Potential disadvantages of internal evaluators
- evaluators could be threatened or tempted to alter results
- it may be hard to ensure lack of bias in internal evaluators
- time must be taken during training to make certain there is awareness of power bestowed
- professional stakeholders may doubt competence of evaluators

Is the role of 'expert' a benefit or detriment?

Administrations that elect to conduct an internal evaluation must consider all of the organizational change which becomes necessary in order to make such an appraisal of services and care worthwhile. By selecting certain staff members to conduct the evaluation, leadership is conveying a message of faith in the observational skills and work ethic of these people. As they see the power of the information they have collected, they may come to see themselves as 'expert'. Other staff may reinforce this divide in the feedback process as they begin to defer to their peers in all care-related matters. Perceptions of how things truly are in the setting may become distorted, and there may be a sense that no further progress needs to be made on the part of observer (Innes 2003).

The key then is to try to determine: how can facilities get the knowledge of an expert without the observable presence of that expert? This question holds implications for organizational change.

Other organizations are emerging with similar values and beliefs. Certain parties in the new culture of care posit that it matters less where the evaluators come from (internal versus external) than where the cultural climate of the setting lies. Perhaps internal evaluation of care can be validated if this evaluation is also evaluated.

Does internal evaluation increase chances that results will be considered and even implemented? Any organizations that have had any degree of success using evaluative methods to improve the quality of care have known of the importance of clinical leadership, of individuals who ask 'What is the intention of this evaluation of the dementia care setting? What is our motivation for undergoing it? What will we do with the results when we get them?' (Brooker and Rogers 2001, p.16).

Conclusions about internal versus external evaluation

Action research can tie the best components of external and internal evaluation together for the most favourable result. Stake (2004) suggests that action research can stem from both an individual and an institutional effort to evaluate and understand. Action research is the study of not only one's practice but of oneself. It asks the individual to consider questions such as: 'What are my predispositions?' 'What are my biases?'

In certain conditions, a skilfully combined use of both internal and external evaluation can have a bimodal benefit. As in the case with Parker (1999) and his students, an academic body may create a contract with a local dementia setting and choose to conduct an evaluation as a field placement of sorts for its social work students. As a result, a facility will get sincere results from enthusiastic evaluators. At the same time desirable evaluative qualities, such as learning how to enable staff to problem-solve many of their own daily dilemmas, could be potentially instilled in insightful students (Parker 1999).

Reflection is key to the success of an evaluator in his role. Each individual must check in with himself to consider the strength of his convictions, the degree of flexibility and fairness he is offering – is it enough? To construct an evaluation of any worth, the participants in gathering data must consider their skills to be of worth as well (Stake 2004).

Regardless of whether the evaluation is pursued internally or externally, Rossi and Freeman (1993) suggest that it is the evaluator's responsibility to cultivate clear understandings of their roles with staff. To a certain degree this requires a garnering of respect. In the end, evaluators must not lose sight of the idea that Esterberg (2002) notes, 'the outcome of research should be useful, aimed at improving the lives of those who are the subject of research. The most desirable outcome of action research is social change' (p.135).

References

Alzheimer's Association (2005) *Campaign for Quality Residential Care: Dementia Care Practice Recommendations for Assisted Living Residences and Nursing Homes.* www.alz.org.

Baker, C.J. and Edwards, P.A. (2002) 'The missing link: benchmarking person-centered care.' *Journal of Dementia Care 10*, 6, 22–23.

Baker, C.J., Edwards, P.A. and Packer, T. (2003a) 'Crucial impact of the world surrounding care.' *Journal of Dementia Care 11*, 3, 16–18.

Baker, C.J., Edwards, P.A. and Packer, T. (2003b) '"You say you deliver person-centred care? Prove it!"' *Journal of Dementia Care 11*, 4, 18–20.

Black, B.S., Rabins, P.V. and Kasper, J.D. (2000) *Alzheimer's Disease Related Quality of Life Users Manual.* Baltimore: DEMeasure.

Bradford Dementia Group (1997) *Evaluating Dementia Care: The DCM Method* (Seventh edition). Bradford: University of Bradford.

Brod, M., Stewart, A.L., Sands, L. and Walton, P. (1999) 'Conceptualization and measurement of quality of life in dementia: the Dementia Quality of Life instrument (DQoL).' *The Gerontologist 39*, 25–35.

Brooker, D. (2002) 'Dementia Care Mapping: a look at its past, present and future.' *Journal of Dementia Care 10*, 3, 33–36.

Brooker, D. and Rogers, L. (eds) (2001) *Dementia Care Mapping (DCM) Think Tank Transcripts.* Bradford: University of Bradford, Bradford Dementia Group.

Doyle, C. (1992) 'Evaluation of innovative dementia programmes: a short review.' Paper presented to the Australian Association of Gerontology.

Edelman, P., Fulton, B.R., Kuhn, D. and Chang, C.H. (2005) 'A comparison of three methods of measuring dementia-specific quality of life: perspectives of residents, staff and observers.' *The Gerontologist 45*, Special Issue, 27–36.

Esterberg, K.G. (2002) *Qualitative Methods in Social Research.* London: McGraw-Hill Publications.

Innes, A. (2003) 'Using Dementia Care Mapping data for care planning purposes.' In A. Innes (ed.) *Dementia Care Mapping: Applications Across Cultures.* Baltimore: Health Professions Press.

Jennings, B. (2000) 'A life greater than the sum of its sensations: ethics, dementia and quality of life.' In S.M. Albert and R.G. Logsdon (eds) *Assessing Quality of Life in Alzheimer's Disease.* New York: Springer Publishing Company.

Kitwood, T. (1997) *Dementia Reconsidered: The Person Comes First.* Buckingham: Open University Press.

Krause, D. (1996) *Effective Program Evaluation.* Chicago: Nelson-Hall Publications.

Lawton, M.P. (2001) 'Quality of care and quality of life in dementia units.' In L.S. Noelker and Z. Harel (eds) *Linking Quality of Long-Term Care and Quality of Life.* New York: Springer Publishing Company.

Logsdon, R.G., Gibbons, L.E., McCurry, S.M. and Teri, L. (2000) 'Quality of life in Alzheimer's disease: patient and caregiver reports.' In S. Albert and R.G. Logsdon (eds) *Assessing Quality of Life in Alzheimer's Disease.* New York: Springer Publishing Company.

Lustbader, W. (2001) 'The pioneer challenge: a radical change in the culture of nursing homes.' In L.S. Noelker and Z. Harel (eds) *Linking Quality of Long-Term Care and Quality of Life.* New York: Springer Publishing Company.

Muller-Hergl, C. (2003) 'A critical reflection of Dementia Care Mapping in Germany.' In A. Innes (ed.) *Dementia Care Mapping: Applications Across Cultures.* Baltimore: Health Professions Press.

Parker, J. (1999) 'Education and learning for the evaluation of dementia care: the perceptions of social workers in training.' *Education and Training 14*, 3, 297–314.

Posavac, E.L. and Carey, R.G. (1992) *Program Evaluation: Methods and Case Studies.* Englewood Cliffs, New Jersey: Prentice Hall.

Rabins, P.V., Lyketsos, C.G. and Steel, C.D. (1999) *Practical Dementia Care.* Oxford: Oxford University Press.

Rossi, P.H. and Freeman, H.E. (1993) *Evaluation: A Systematic Approach.* Newbury Park, California: Sage.

Sloane, P.D., Zimmerman, S., Williams, C.S., Reed, P.S., Gill, K.S. and Preisser, J.S. (2005) 'Evaluating the quality of life of long-term care residents with dementia.' *The Gerontologist 45*, Special Issue, 37–49.

Stake, R.E. (2004) *Standards-Based and Responsive Evaluation.* Thousand Oaks, California: Sage.

Twigg, J. (2000) *Bathing – The Body and Community Care.* London and New York: Routledge.

Walker, E. and Dewar, B. with Dewing, J. and Pritchard, E. (2001) *An Evaluation of Day Care Services for People with Dementia from the Perspective of Major Stakeholders.* Edinburgh: Centre for the Older Person's Agenda, Queen Margaret University College.

Chapter 4

The Policy Context for Evaluating Dementia Care

Louise McCabe

This chapter explores the links between policy and evaluation. It begins by looking in some detail at policy that is directly concerned with evaluating health and care services. The type of evaluation processes that are most closely influenced by health and social care policy are the regulation and inspection of services. The chapter includes a brief history of the ever-changing policy of regulation of both health and social care before looking at current legislation and its operation. Further detail is given on the standards of care for the different health and care services that these policies promote, before discussion on how these standards relate to concepts of good quality care. The chapter covers policy and selected care standards in Scotland, England, Wales and Northern Ireland. It discusses the advantages and disadvantages of the type of evaluation involved in the processes of regulation and inspection of services and considers how this compares to other evaluation processes. In conclusion, I reflect on whether service providers are influenced or guided by policy when they engage in evaluations of their services and how evaluations may in turn influence policy and change.

Before the discussion on regulation of services it is important to be clear about what services are being discussed. Cheston, Bender and Byatt (2000) state that people with dementia can experience a wide range of NHS, social and voluntary services. They may have a service career wherein they move through a range of services over time and service changes may be rapid. Therefore, to evaluate dementia care as a whole it is necessary to look at many different services. Some of the key services used by people with dementia include residential and nursing homes for older people and increasingly domiciliary care services. In the literature there has been a greater focus on residential care as a site for evaluation than home care services which have received little attention (Parahoo, Campbell and Scoltock 2002).

Over the past 10 to 20 years there have been changes in where people with dementia live and therefore a change in the types of services and professionals that they utilize and which therefore need to be regulated and evaluated. More people with dementia are living in the community with more focus on home care services. Changes in the client groups in care homes mean that managers have to re-evaluate the tasks of different types of staff; there has also been a blurring of the line between residential and nursing homes (O'Kell 1995). There have been changes in which sectors provide care and who is responsible for the regulation of services. The statutory sector now has responsibility for the regulation of services provided by voluntary, private and statutory organizations. As a consequence statutory organizations now take a lesser role in providing services but are more involved in contracting and commissioning services as well as regulation. Regulation of services has various aims but the main one is to ensure the quality of services. This is both to improve the current situation for people with dementia and to improve future care for people with dementia. A recent history of regulating care is given below followed by a discussion of the current policy context of regulation in the four countries of the UK.

Regulating care for people with dementia

This section looks at the recent history of the regulation of care in different parts of the UK. Regulation has a complex history with many different systems for inspecting services and applying standards to care. However, there has been little actual legislative change for many years (Day, Klein and Redmayne 1996). Until recently, the Registered Homes Act 1984 provided for regulation of nursing and residential homes for older people

(O'Kell 1995). A wide variety of quality assurance systems have been developed and used in residential and nursing homes in recent years (O'Kell 1995).

The National Health Service and Community Care Act 1990 (Department of Health 1990) gave local authorities the lead in inspecting both statutory and independent care services. It also made some important changes to existing inspection and regulation systems by introducing lay assessors into the inspection teams and giving teams semi-autonomous status. Inspection reports also became public documents allowing anyone to access their content. Following the NHS and Community Care Act each part of the UK developed their own system for regulation.

In England there are 107 different local authorities and before recent policy changes, discussed below, each had their own approach to regulation and their own interpretation of ambiguous policy guidelines. This led to inconsistencies in the frequency of inspections and in the methods used for evaluating services, particularly residential and nursing homes (Day *et al.* 1996; O'Kell 1995). In the Registered Homes Act 1984 terms such as 'adequacy' and 'sufficiency' were left for local authorities to interpret and produce local guidance (Day *et al.* 1996; O'Kell 1995). For example, some local authorities insisted on all single rooms in homes while others required as few as 20 per cent (Day *et al.* 1996). Assessment of quality in residential homes has focused on measuring management and staff quality with very little focus on individual care plans and residents (Challis, Carpenter and Traske 1996). There were problems of inconsistency caused by too many different inspection groups (Day *et al.* 1996). Previously in Scotland, the 32 local authorities and 12 mainland health boards carried out regulation and inspection duties. Similar to England, each had a slightly different system and operated to different standards (Care Commission 2005). These regulations also did not cover all care services (Scottish Parliament 2001b).

The complexity of the systems hindered the aims of regulatory bodies and in turn the quality of services provided for people with dementia. The lack of consistency across and between areas has prevented the delivery of consistently good quality services. There appear to be too many people involved in these processes and no clear pathway for service providers or service users.

Since the late 1990s there had been increasing calls to change the way care services were regulated. A need was perceived for a national body, independent of local authorities and health boards, which would take the lead in regulating health and care services. The report of the Royal Commission on Long Term Care for Older People identified a need for what they called a 'national care commission' (Royal Commission on Long Term Care 1999). The Joseph Rowntree Foundation (JRF) also called for a national system for regulating and registering nursing and residential homes (JRF 1996). Two pieces of research commissioned by the JRF in the mid-1990s involved consultation with directors of social services and inspection team heads. These groups also supported the idea of a single national regulatory body (Day *et al.* 1996; O'Kell 1995).

In Scotland the system of regulation was criticized for its lack of independence as local authorities and health boards might both provide and regulate the same services (Scottish Executive 1999). It was also criticized for a lack of consistency with differing standards applied across Scotland and a lack of integration for example between nursing and residential care which may be provided in the same building but have different regulatory bodies (Scottish Executive 1999). Some of the regulatory policy in Scotland came from as far back as 1938. Independently run nursing homes were regulated by the Nursing Homes Registration (Scotland) Act 1938 until the recent changes described below (Scottish Executive 2005). Home care services had been largely exempt from regulation and inspection and these issues are addressed in the new regulations (Pearson and Riddell 2003).

A report published in Scotland strongly criticizes standards developed prior to the 2000s. The standards were based on eight values: privacy, dignity, respect, choice, independence, rights, fulfilment and safety. However, in practice little attention was paid to these (Pearson and Riddell 2003). A review of the regulatory process found that inspection teams focused more on practical concerns and the physical environment (Pearson and Riddell 2003). There were significant differences in the ways in which health boards inspected nursing homes and social service units inspected residential homes. Inspection of nursing homes focuses on specific nursing tasks and regimes with little attention paid to residents' social needs (Pearson and Riddell 2003). This report also examined the inclusion of user views in inspection reports and found this to be significantly lacking for most service users including older people and people with mental health problems (Pearson and Riddell 2003). Despite significant numbers of residents being people with dementia little mention of them was made in relation to gathering user views. For example in Edinburgh and Lothian it was simply stated that people with dementia were unable to express their views about the homes they lived in (Pearson and Riddell 2003, p.28). When user and staff views were included, their comments were summarized and given in brief (Pearson and Riddell 2003).

Important changes to legislation influencing registration and regulation of services took place in the early 2000s. The key piece of legislation in England and Wales was the Care Standards Act 2000 (Department of Health 2000) and in Scotland, the Regulation of Care (Scotland) Act 2001 (Scottish Parliament 2001b). These pieces of legislation came into effect in early 2002. During this period of change things were confused and muddled. Many inspectors moved from old to new systems and care home owners were busy trying to meet new standards (O'Kell 2002). These changes led to the current situation in the UK.

Current policy regulating care in the UK

In England and Wales two major pieces of legislation shape the regulation of health and care services, the Care Standards Act 2000 and the Health and Social Care (Community Health and Standards) Act 2003 (Department of Health 2003). The Care Standards Act came into effect from April 2002 and laid the framework for the establishment of a new regulatory body, the 'National Care Standards Commission' (NCSC). The NCSC was responsible for the regulation, registration and setting of standards for a wide range of services. For people with dementia the most relevant services included: residential care, nursing homes, domiciliary support services, nurses' agencies and independent medical agencies. The Care Standards Act also set up the General Social Care Council and Care Council which makes provision for the registration, regulation and training of social workers. The NCSC also had responsibility for supporting service users and advising ministers. The Care Standards Act also specifies national minimum standards for those services it regulates. The standards for relevant services are discussed in more detail later. Standards cover issues such as room size, ratio of bathrooms, size of living group and aspects of the care provided in different services. The Care Standards Act also set out guidelines for new bodies to be responsible for the inspection and regulation of services: the Commission for Healthcare Audit and Inspection (CHAI) and the Commission for Social Care Inspection (CSCI). The Health and Social Care (Community Health and Standards) Act 2003 then established these two regulatory bodies in 2004. They replace the NCSC and the Commission for Health Improvement and form two separate bodies, one for health care, and one for social care.

The CHAI covers England and has some functions in Wales while other aspects of health care are the responsibility of the Welsh Assembly. The CSCI's remit is restricted to England only. Box 4.1 lists the main functions of the CSCI and the following section gives some detail on its aims. Although CHAI and CSCI are exclusive to England, their aims and philosophy reflect the new approach to inspection and regulation adopted across the UK.

The CSCI combines the work formerly done by the Social Services Inspectorate, the Social Services Inspectorate/Audit Commission joint review team and the NCSC. The CSCI aims to allow a more rational, integrated system of social care inspection and regulation (CSCI 2004a). The CSCI takes on an intelligence role as well as that of inspecting and regulating. They can also take action when services are failing (CSCI 2004b).

The CSCI put a strong emphasis on user involvement, giving their first priority as 'putting people first – taking more notice of the views of those who actually use social care' (CSCI 2004c, p.7). It is interesting to note that when setting out why they regulate services they give the reason that many older people in residential care may experience confusion, depression or dementia (CSCI 2004c, p.8). This seems to indicate that people with dementia are seen as an important group of users of social care

---

Box 4.1 The main functions of the Commission for Social Care Inspection (CSCI)

- To carry out inspections of all social care organizations – public, private and voluntary – against national standards and publish inspection reports
- To register services meeting standards
- To inspect and assess 'value for money' of council social services
- To publish an annual report on the state of social care
- To validate statistics on social care
- To publish ratings for social services authorities

(CSCI 2004a, 2005)

---

services. The CSCI acknowledges many of the shortfalls of previous and current inspection systems such as too much time 'ticking boxes' and not enough time talking to those who use care services (CSCI 2004c). They are currently implementing changes to rectify these shortcomings.

The CHAI, also known as the Healthcare Commission, claims to put the experiences of patients at the core of everything they do. All outputs from the commission are available to the public. Similar to the CSCI the CHAI is also an amalgamation of different organizations. The CHAI should offer a more streamlined service with the aim of helping service users to access and understand information (CHAI 2005). Box 4.2 lists the main functions of CHAI.

More recently, the Department of Health has recommended further changes. The Green Paper *Independence, Well-being and Choice* (Department of Health 2005) sets out a vision for the future of social care for adults in England. This document recommends the merging of CSCI and CHAI by 2008 due to the increasing joint work between adult health and social care. This area of policy continues to change.

Within the UK each constituent country has different regulatory bodies and is developing its own standards and inspection methods. In Wales the Care Standards Inspectorate for Wales (CSIW) is responsible for

---

Box 4.2 The main functions of the Commission for Healthcare Audit and Inspection (CHAI)

- To encourage improvement in health care
- To inspect the management, provision and quality of health care services – public, private and voluntary
- To investigate serious service failures
- To publish annual performance ratings for all NHS organizations
- To carry out an independent review function for NHS complaints

(CHAI 2005)

---

the inspection and regulation of social care services and health care services run by voluntary and private organizations (CSIW 2005). The CSIW is bound by the same statutory framework as the CSCI and fulfils many similar functions. It has four specific elements to its work, registration, inspection, complaints and enforcement, and is responsible for setting national minimum standards for care services in Wales. It is operationally independent from the National Assembly of Wales. Again, this organization stresses that its first priority is to service users (CSIW 2005).

In Scotland changes to the regulatory framework took place at the same time. A series of consultation papers commissioned by the Scottish Parliament between 1998 and 2001 concerned issues about social services and private and voluntary health care services (Scottish Parliament 2001a). Many of these consultation papers related to the regulation of health and social care and to the development of care standards for different services. These led to the passing of the Regulation of Care (Scotland) Act 2001. This Act established a new independent body to regulate care services in Scotland, the Scottish Commission for the Regulation of Care, known as the Care Commission (Scottish Parliament 2001a). The Care Commission is responsible for the regulation and registration of social care services plus independent, voluntary and private health care services (Scottish Parliament 2001a). The Regulation of Care (Scotland) Act also established a body, called the Scottish Social Services Council, to regulate social service workers and to promote and regulate their education and training (Scottish Parliament 2001a).

The Care Commission is similar to the CSIW with the same four elements to its function: inspection, registration, complaints and enforcement (Care Commission 2005). The Care Commission will ensure that regulations are applied consistently across Scotland and will report to the Scottish Parliament on the provision and quality of care services in Scotland (Care Commission 2005). The Care Commission states that it will prioritize the 'dignity, choice and safety' of the service users (Care Commission 2005).

In Northern Ireland the Health and Personal Social Services (Quality, Improvement and Regulation) (Northern Ireland) Order 2003 makes provision for the Department of Health, Social Services and Public Safety to develop minimum standards of care (DHSSPS Online 2005). The Health and Personal Social Services Regulation and Improvement Authority (HPSSRIA) will use these standards to regulate and improve a wide range of health and social care services. This authority started work in April 2005. In addition a Standards Development Task Group has been set up and is currently developing and consulting on various sets of standards (DHSSPS Online 2005).

Each of the four countries of the UK appears to be at different stages of very similar processes. An independent national body will undertake inspections and develop standards for a wide range of health and social care services in all four countries. Northern Ireland is currently in the earlier stages of developing their regulatory systems while England has already redesigned its system for the second time. Each of the different organizations stresses a commitment to service users and the importance of direct consultation with them. This reflects wider policy recognition of the importance of service user views and an apparent commitment to provide quality services. These organizations all aim to promote good quality care. Their understandings of this concept are illustrated by the care standards they develop for different services and different service user groups.

Key to people with dementia and their carers are services such as residential care, domiciliary care agencies and hospital care, both acute and long-term. The following section looks at some of the standards drawn up by the different countries for services such as residential care for older people and domiciliary care agencies. The following discussion explores the depth and focus of the regulatory and evaluation processes they frame.

Standards of care

Closely linked with the process of regulation are the standards used by the different agencies to judge and evaluate different services (known in England as National Minimum Standards and in Scotland as National Care Standards). These set out both structural and environmental standards as well as promoting a particular philosophy of care. In England, the standards also highlight important outcomes for service users such as choice of home; lifestyle and personal development; complaints and protection; staffing and management. The new standards, following the Care Standards Act 2000, become mandatory in 2007. The Healthcare Commission in England publishes standards on a range of topics grouped into seven key areas: safety, clinical and cost effectiveness, governance, patient focus, accessible and responsive care, care environment, and amenities and public health (CHAI 2005).

Within a review of the new standards for independently run residential care in England some people consulted felt that the National Minimum Standards concentrated more on structure and process issues and did not really improve on those within the Registered Homes Act 1984 (O'Kell 2002). There is still a need to incorporate a stronger focus on outcomes. Others felt that the new standards were 'clear, visible and unequivocal' (O'Kell 2002, p.42).

In Wales the CSIW is still in the process of developing national minimum standards for many services but some are already published such as those for domiciliary care agencies. These standards came into force in March 2004 and cover user and carer issues as well as standards for management and staff providing domiciliary care. It sets out a definition for personal care and regulates only services that provide this (Welsh

Assembly Government 2004). Standards set out how a person should be assessed, what information should be provided, the standard and philosophy of care provided and guidelines for hiring staff.

In Northern Ireland minimum care standards are still in the development or consultation stages. A range of standards are being drawn up including those for domiciliary care services, day care settings, residential homes, nursing homes and nursing agencies. These are similar to the range of standards drawn up in the other parts of the UK.

The new standards in Scotland have been developed in consultation with service users and their carers through a body called the National Care Standards Committee (Whatling 2003). However, a review of the consultation process highlighted that not enough service users, carers and representatives of minority ethnic groups had been involved (Whatling 2003). Similar to the other countries of the UK, Scotland has also developed a range of national minimum standards for different services.

Aims and philosophy of current systems of regulation

Underpinning the regulatory and inspection processes and the national minimum care standards is a philosophy of 'good quality care' which the different organizations are trying to promote. An apparent focus on user and carer involvement is apparent in the development of care standards, and the importance of user views is stressed within inspections. A focus on user and care involvement has been increasingly apparent in policy since the National Health Service and Community Care Act 1990. This Act talks about and promotes choice and user and carer involvement in care planning (Cheston *et al.* 2000). Cheston *et al.* (2000) emphasize how successive governments have promoted the principle of user involvement in services. As discussed above, service users and their carers have been involved to some extent in the development of national minimum care standards in each of the four countries of the UK. However, as highlighted by Whatling (2003), there could have been more involvement by these groups.

There has also been a more recent focus on outcomes for service users. By asking service users and their carers about service outcomes it is possible to evaluate that service. Pritchard and Dewing (2001) discuss a very specific approach to caring for people with dementia and evaluate their programme by asking users and their carers about outcomes. They stress that there have been few studies evaluating dementia services which involve users and carers in the evaluation. A report by the Joseph Rowntree Foundation (JRF 2003), however, found that it can be difficult for users to focus on outcomes when services are poor.

The following discussion focuses on two sets of standards: the National Care Standard 'Care at Home' (Scottish Executive 2005) and the National Service Framework for Older People (Department of Health 2001). Each of these documents presents a concept of good care and places values on different elements of care services, both environmental and social. The standards reflect current thinking within policy on the provision of good quality care for people with dementia.

All Scottish Executive National Care Standards are based around six principles: 'dignity, privacy, choice, safety, realising potential and equality and diversity' (Scottish Executive 2005, p.3). These principles are there to ensure the promotion of quality, person-centred services. These are noble aims and the principles fit with concepts such as Kitwood's person-centred care (Kitwood 1997) and other social approaches to working with people with dementia. It is, however, difficult to balance between the sometimes conflicting issues raised by different principles. The obvious pair might be choice and safety; there are often dilemmas about promoting choice while reducing risk.

The National Care Standard 'Care at Home' (revised March 2005) also promotes equality but in the introduction goes on to single children out for special attention. The standards highlight that children's wishes may be different from parents and family members but that is also true for most people including people with dementia whose wishes are often compromised. Looking at the standards overall they appear to promote person-centred services focusing on individual choices and views. However, people with dementia are also compromised by the standards. In Standard Three in relation to a service user moving between services, reference is made to competency and consent and the phrase 'if you are able to give it [consent]' is used. This passing reference to consent appears to indicate that whether someone is able to give consent or not is a simple issue. However, as dementia practitioners and researchers, we know this is not the case.

The National Service Framework for Older People similarly appears to promote person-centred care and services for older people and includes the added aim of 'rooting out' age discrimination. Standard Seven relates to mental health in older people and includes people with dementia. This standard appears to support many of the principles of person-centred care for people with dementia. For example, Standard Seven, Section 11 talks about choice in activities and matching these to needs and preferences; it notes the importance of a good environment with 'good quality design, lighting, colour contrast and access'. However, in the discussion specific to dementia a medical approach is taken regarding diagnosis and treatment.

These different standards illustrate the complexity of the situation regarding regulation and evaluation of services for people with dementia. There is conflict between different goals and aspirations, conflict between choice for the service users and budgetary restraints for service providers. It would be a wonderful world if all the components of all standards were practically achievable.

From the above discussion it appears that formal approaches to evaluating services through inspection and regulation have positive values and aims. User involvement, choice, empowerment and outcomes for service users are all concepts used in discussions on good quality care. The issue for regulators is the relationship between these values and aims and the actual impact policy has on services. The practical guidelines offered in some standards such as room sizes and occupancy and staff ratios are concrete ways in which standards can improve care for people with dementia. In contrast concepts such as empowerment and choice are harder to pin down. Standards provide a structured set of guidelines against which services are measured. These standards ensure fairness and consistency across service providers and allow evaluators to measure effectively and to compare aspects of services. However, this rigidity may also be a disadvantage, as it is difficult to measure how much service users are empowered or how they are offered choices. The links between policy and practice are relatively close and can be clearly seen. This type of evaluation process provides a specific type of information for a specific purpose. The specific purpose of regulation both limits and enhances this approach to evaluation.

Advantages and disadvantages to policy-driven evaluation processes

The formal nature of regulation and its roots in policy mean there is an inherent structure and bureaucracy to the inspection system. There is a need for consistency between different inspections to fit with set standards making the system rigid and difficult to adapt to particular services. There is a need to employ different techniques to effectively evaluate services for people with different levels of cognitive ability and from different social groups, such as minority ethnic groups, and formal inspection processes may fail to do this (Cheston *et al.* 2000). Care standards may also over-simplify the care and support offered by services and practitioners (Munro 2004). Care and support services are by nature complex and individual and it can be difficult to assess exactly what aspects of a service are most important for service users; it is difficult to define quality (McHale 2003). For services for people with dementia the term 'person-centred care' is often used as a descriptor of good quality care. However, there is little consensus in the literature on what person-centred care actually looks like or what the term means to service users (Innes, Macpherson and McCabe 2006). Inspections are made more complex by the huge diversity of health and social care services and the interface between these bureaucracies (McHale 2003).

There may be conflict between service outcomes and user outcomes. For many services there is tension between the needs of funders or commissioners and the service users themselves. There is an increasing demand for service providers and professionals to be accountable and transparent (Munro 2004). For local authority services they need to please both the taxpayers funding the services and the service users. These groups will have very different agendas and possibly different ideas about what makes a good service. Similarly, care homes run by private companies need to satisfy investors and service users. An inspection becomes, therefore, something between an audit and an evaluation of good care.

One way of addressing these problems is through the presence of lay assessors within the inspection teams. Lay assessors provide an unbiased, in some ways naïve, perspective. Historically some inspection teams have used, and still use, lay assessors (Wright 2005). Research has found that they can strengthen the work of inspection teams as they tend to spend more time talking to service users and present a less formal face to the inspection process (Wright 2005). Inspection team members may be caught up in the paperwork and policy of inspection, and lay assessors may therefore add valuable information for the inspection. Wright (2005) found that lay assessors take different approaches to the inspection process but in general spent time talking to service users and observing their interactions and behaviour. This second part was seen as important in care homes where people with dementia lived (Wright 2005).

There are also many advantages to such systems of evaluation. The current systems involve external inspection. This type of evaluation is important for a number of reasons, as highlighted within *Independence, Well-being and Choice, Our Vision for the Future of Social Care for Adults in England* (Department of Health 2005):

- People using services are often vulnerable and may be unable to speak for themselves.

- It is difficult for users and carers to assess quality before choosing services and difficult to change services if they are found to be poor.

- People are increasingly using their own resources to pay for social care.

They ensure that inspection and regulation extend to a wide range of the services used by people with dementia. The structured and formalized nature of inspection ensures consistency of approach across different services and different areas ensuring that services meet set standards. They help to ensure a minimum standard but also help to promote higher standards and motivate service providers to improve.

Conclusion

The problems and issues discussed above with these types of evaluation highlight the ways in which they differ from other types of evaluation. They are designed to apply across a wide variety of situations and their aim is to ensure a minimum standard of care across different services and locations. Care standards are designed for groups of services and, therefore, they cannot accurately predict the needs of all service users. Inspection processes are also undertaken for a number of reasons and for a number of audiences; funders and commissioners as well as service users need to be satisfied. These types of evaluation process do not provide the detailed and specific pictures that would be obtained using other evaluation techniques. Some bigger organizations, such as health boards, do use detailed evaluation techniques such as Dementia Care Mapping (Brooker *et al.* 1998) and the Positive Response Schedule (Hadley, Brown and Smith 1999). These evaluations are used to support the work of different organizations but it is not clear from the research how these relate to regulatory processes going on at the same time. It is clear that these more complex and time-consuming techniques could not feasibly be used to the same extent as current inspection processes.

This chapter has illustrated the manner in which policy changes impact on regulation and inspection processes and in turn on services. The language of recent policy, that is the way 'good quality services' are described in policy, shapes the aims of evaluators. The evaluation processes discussed here show a clear link between policy and evaluation and illustrate the ways in which changes in policy have influenced formal evaluation systems and their aims. As a result policy also influences change in services. Service providers and commissioners are influenced by policy rhetoric and through evaluation processes may implement change. The new regulatory bodies have powers to implement changes in services that fail to meet the given standards. This is a real advantage to this type of evaluation. In this way policy aims directly influence the experience of service users. The focus on service user views may also lead to their influence on policy through feedback during the processes of inspection and regulation. However, it is important to remember that there are many disadvantages to these types of evaluation and these limitations will limit their ability to promote and bring about positive change.

References

Brooker, D., Foster, N., Banner, A., Payne, M. and Jackson, L. (1998) 'The efficacy of Dementia Care Mapping as an audit tool: report of a 3-year British NHS evaluation.' *Aging and Mental Health 2*, 1, 60–70.

Care Commission (2005) *About Us.* Available at: www.carecommission.com/aboutus/index.php. Accessed February 2005.

CHAI (2005) *Healthcare Commission FAQs.* Available at: www.chai.org.uk. Accessed February 2005.

Challis, D., Carpenter, I. and Traske, K. (1996) *Towards a National Standard Assessment Instrument for Residential and Nursing Home Care.* Kent: Personal Social Services Research Unit.

Cheston, R., Bender, M. and Byatt, S. (2000) 'Involving people who have dementia in the evaluation of services: a review.' *Journal of Mental Health 9*, 5, 471–479.

CSCI (2004a) *The Commission and its Work with Independent Providers.* London: CSCI.

CSCI (2004b) *Role and Responsibilities.* London: CSCI.

CSCI (2004c) *Inspecting for Better Lives (Modernising the Regulation of Social Care).* London: CSCI.

CSCI (2005) *CSCI or CHAI?* London: CSCI.

CSIW (2005) *About Us.* Available at: www.csiw.wales.gov.uk/fe/default.asp?n1=2. Accessed February 2005.

Day, P., Klein, R. and Redmayne, S. (1996) *Why Regulate? Regulating Care for Elderly People.* Bristol: The Policy Press.

Department of Health (1990) *National Health Service and Community Care Act 1990.* Available at: www.hmso.gov.uk/acts/acts1990/Ukpga_19900019_en_1.htm. Accessed Febuary 2005.

Department of Health (2000) *Care Standards Act 2000.* Available at: www.hmso.gov.uk/acts/acts2000/20000014.htm. Accessed February 2005.

Department of Health (2001) *National Service Framework for Older People.* London: HMSO. Available at: www.dh.gov.uk/assetRoot/04/07/12/83/04071283.pdf. Accessed Febuary 2005.

Department of Health (2003) *Explanatory Notes to Health and Social Care (Community Health and Standards) Act 2003.* Available at: www.hmso.gov.uk/acts/en2003/2003en43.htm. Accessed February 2005.

Department of Health (2005) *Independence, Well-being and Choice, Our Vision for the Future of Social Care for Adults in England.* London: HMSO. Available at: www.dh.gov.uk/assetRoot/04/10/64/78/04106478.pdf. Accessed Febuary 2005.

DHSSPS Online (2005) *Care Standards FAQs.* Available at: www.dhsspsni.gov.uk/governance-carefaqs. Accessed February 2005.

Hadley, C., Brown, S. and Smith, A. (1999) 'Evaluating interventions for people with severe dementia: using the Positive Response Schedule.' *Aging and Mental Health 3*, 3, 234–240.

Innes, A., Macpherson, S. and McCabe, L. (2006) *Promoting Person Centred Care at the Frontline.* York: Joseph Rowntree Foundation.

JRF (1996) *Unified Registration and National Regulation Systems Urged for Care Homes.* JRF Press Release. Available at: www.jrf.org.uk/pressroom/releases/021196.asp. Accessed February 2005.

JRF (2003) *Service Users' Own Definitions of Quality Outcomes.* York: Joseph Rowntree Foundation. Available at: www.jrf.org.uk/knowledge/findings/socialcare/673.asp. Accessed February 2005.

Kitwood, T. (1997) *Dementia Reconsidered: The Person Comes First.* Buckingham: Open University Press.

McHale, J. (2003) 'Standards, quality and accountability – the NHS and mental health: a case for joined-up thinking?' *Journal of Social Welfare and Family Law 25,* 4, 369–382.

Munro, E. (2004) 'The impact of audit on social work practice.' *British Journal of Social Work 34,* 1075–1095.

O'Kell, S. (1995) *Care Standards in the Residential Care Sector.* York: Joseph Rowntree Foundation.

O'Kell, S. (2002) *The Independent Care Homes Sector.* York: Joseph Rowntree Foundation.

Parahoo, K., Campbell, A. and Scoltock, C. (2002) 'An evaluation of a domiciliary respite service for younger people with dementia.' *Journal of Evaluation in Clinical Practice 8,* 4, 377–385.

Pearson, C. and Riddell, S. (2003) *Standards of Care and the Regulation of Care Services in Scotland.* Edinburgh: The Stationery Office.

Pritchard, E. and Dewing, J. (2001) 'A multi-method evaluation of an independent dementia care service and its approach.' *Aging and Mental Health 5,* 1, 63–72.

Royal Commission on Long Term Care (1999) *With Respect to Old Age: Long Term Care – Rights and Responsibilities.* The Report of the Royal Commission on Long Term Care, Cm 4192-I. London: The Stationery Office.

Scottish Executive (1999) *Regulating Care and the Social Services Workforce.* Available at: www.scotland.gov.uk/library2/doc10/rcsw-01.asp. Accessed February 2005.

Scottish Executive (2005) *Regulating the Independent Healthcare Sector.* Publications Online. Available at: www.scotland.gov.uk/library3/health/rihs-01.asp. Accessed February 2005.

Scottish Parliament (2001a) *Explanatory Notes to Regulation of Care (Scotland) Act.* Available at: www.scotland-legislation.hmso.gov.uk/legislation/scotland/en2001/2001en08.htm. Accessed February 2005.

Scottish Parliament (2001b) *Regulation of Care (Scotland) Act.* Available at: www.scotland-legislation.hmso.gov.uk/legislation/scotland/acts2001/20010008.htm. Accessed February 2005.

Welsh Assembly Government (2004) *National Minimum Standards for Domiciliary Care Agencies in Wales.* Available at: www.wales.gov.uk/subisocialpolicycarestandards/content/regulations/dom-care-wales-e.pdf. Accessed Febuary 2005.

Whatling, R. (2003) *Evaluation of the National Care Standards Consultations.* Edinburgh: The Stationery Office.

Wright, F. (2005) 'Lay assessors and care home inspections: is there a future?' *British Journal of Social Work 35,* 1093–1106.

PART TWO

Evaluating Dementia Care

Practicalities and Reflections

Chapter 5

Evaluating Technology for Dementia Care

Alison Bowes

The potential of technology

In recent years, new electronic technologies capable of supporting older people, including people with dementia, have enjoyed increasing attention, as they have become more sophisticated. These technologies include both telecare systems and stand-alone electronic devices. Announcing an £80 million 'Preventative Technology Grant' for local authorities in England, the Department of Health (2005) suggested that telecare might support more older people to remain at home, cut hospital admissions and improve quality of life for informal carers as well as older people themselves. For government, it could address problems of a diminishing workforce and increased demand for services and also reduce costs. These are radical claims. Yet the evidence base for them remains limited, and in particular, benefits for people with dementia have been little researched.

Alongside the undoubted beneficial impact of new technologies, some commentators highlight potential problems, which may be especially significant for people with dementia. These include the potential for telecare to promote a rejuvenated medical model of dementia, detracting from recent headway made in promoting a disability model (Fisk 2001, p.120). Also, the tendency for a focus on risk resulting in new technology becoming a new form of restraint, watching the person with dementia for 'risky' behaviour which then precipitates residential care, as they are labelled 'personifications of risk' (Manthorpe 2004, p.148). Finally, an emphasis on surveillance, including electronic monitoring or tagging, potentially carried out without the full consent of the person with dementia (Fisk 2001, p.238).

These contrasting images of the impact of new technologies for people with dementia highlight the need for continuing review of the evidence base, for careful evaluation of the use of new technologies to support people with dementia and their informal carers, and for good practice and potential difficulties to be shared. This chapter reviews the current state of evidence regarding new technologies for people with dementia, and highlights some of the issues which consistently arise, and continue to present challenges for the future.

Evidence so far

Technological developments over recent years have been rapid, and there is an increasing market for electronic devices which can be used as part of care regimes – their use is commonly referred to as 'telecare'. Telecare is related to 'telemedicine', and the two may be used together. Whilst there is some debate in the literature regarding precise definitions of both (for example, May 2005), for the purposes of this chapter 'telecare' refers to electronic systems and/or devices used to support social care. Some devices may be used in people's homes or in care settings as 'stand-alone' items. Examples of these would be electronic clock calendars, which support people with time-orientation difficulties, or devices which can help people manage medication, supporting them to take the correct doses of their medicines at the right times. Both these devices were used in Northamptonshire (Woolham 2006a) and in the ENABLE project (discussed below).

Other devices are used in connection with a system of alarms, connected to a home alert console, with calls usually routed through a call centre. These devices include items such as smoke alarms, heat sensors and fall detectors along with movement or lifestyle monitors, such as MIDAS (Modular Intelligent Domiciliary Alarm System – Fisk 2001). On receiving a call from such a device, a call centre operator uses a protocol normally tailored to the individual to call on an appropriate response to the information received. These 'smart' systems – systems and devices which communicate with one another – can also include assistive devices such as door entry systems, window openers and closers, light operators and so on, all of which can be controlled remotely. Many of the devices can operate passively – that is, they do not require action by a user to raise an alarm or to carry out an action, such as closing curtains when darkness falls. Others require action by the user, such as pressing a button to call for assistance.

By themselves, the devices may be seen as neutral, in that they have potential to be used in a variety of ways, positive or not. However, like all technological developments, they cannot be considered as 'purely' technical, in that all technological innovations occur within a social context and are stimulated by issues perceived within that context. Baldwin (2006) eloquently argues that all technological devices reflect values, as, for example, precise clocks reflect a value attached to knowing and working by precise times.

Barlow (2005) notes that the evidence to date about the use of technology in dementia care has emphasized the context in which telecare has been used, thus promoting 'evidence-informed' practice. He notes the preference of clinical practitioners for 'evidence-based' practice deriving from randomized controlled trials, which, he suggests, are neither practical nor desirable for telecare, a 'complex intervention' (Barlow 2005, p.7) involving a number of interacting components whose individual effects are hard to ascertain.

Much of the evidence about telecare comes from evaluations attached to the development of new technological devices and from mainly small-scale use of these devices in real care situations. Much of the research concerns older people and informal carers generally, and there is relatively little work which specifically considers issues for people with dementia, though other long-term conditions have been the subjects of more systematic evaluations – Barlow (2005) identifies work on diabetes, congestive heart failure and chronic obstructive pulmonary disease (COPD).

Evaluating devices

Several studies have examined particular technological devices and their acceptability for and impact on people using them. Two key recent projects focused specifically on people with dementia are the ENABLE project (ENABLE – Enabling Technologies for People with Dementia – 2005; Hagen *et al.* 2004) and the INDEPENDENT project (Sixsmith 2006).

The ENABLE project took a selection of products designed to support people with dementia in various ways. These included a night and day calendar clock; a cooker cut-off device; a 'picture gramophone', which allowed users to choose music by pressing buttons with pictures on them; a lamp which would automatically switch on if someone got out of bed at night; a picture telephone; a locator for lost items such as keys; a device to remind people to take medicine; and a day planner. The project involved research teams in England, Lithuania, Ireland, Finland and Norway. A selection of the products were tested with service users with dementia and their informal carers in each country, using a series of interviews to ascertain how the devices were being used and people's reactions to them.

Despite very small samples in each country, the ENABLE team developed tools for assessing responses to the items of technology (Hagen *et al.* 2004). In particular, they emphasized the importance of the context in which the person with dementia lived and their informal carers as influential. Although some members of the team felt that some of the research instruments were too complex, and the resulting interviews too long, the protocol nevertheless highlights important issues in considering the impact of technology in dementia care. Importantly, the researchers emphasized that people with dementia were able to contribute directly to the evaluation process.

The project reports, published on the website (www.enable-project.org/), suggest that the devices, especially the clock, were in many cases useful, helping with some of the challenges of daily living presented by having dementia and, in the case of the picture gramophone, offering enjoyment and enhancing quality of life (Topo and Saarikalle 2005). The reports also indicate that people in the early stages of dementia are likely to benefit the most – the researchers suggest that early use of technologies like these is more beneficial, and habits may then be established which can last, even where cognitive functioning later deteriorates.

A major issue which emerged from the ENABLE project concerned the unreliability of some of the devices. Some were quickly found not to be ready for general use – notably the cooker regulator and the locator – and several were withdrawn from use for that reason. The Finnish report (Topo *et al.* 2005, p.42) noted that unreliable products could cause 'stress and harm' for people with dementia and their carers. A second issue concerned cultural differences affecting the operation of the technology. This issue was exemplified by the bed monitor linked to the lamp which did not work in Finnish beds (Topo *et al.* 2005). Other issues were specific to particular devices. The picture gramophone, though receiving a generally positive response, was felt to be time-consuming to set up and therefore less attractive for care workers to use than an ordinary radio or CD player. The telephone was found to be too similar to devices readily available on the open market to be worthwhile developing, and many people were found already to have similar apparatus, which was indeed effective in helping them use the telephone.

The INDEPENDENT project, described by Sixsmith (2006), has as its central focus the promotion of pleasure and enjoyment, shifting attention from the more negative images of care needs and focusing on the development of new devices, rather than using those already available. The research began by working with people with dementia and their carers' own perspectives on their quality of life, using these to identify areas where technology could provide improvements. One emerging area from these data was that of music (Sixsmith and Gibson 2006), significant in many people's lives and a key source of enjoyment. Participants' comments revealed a need for a specific technological device that would allow people to choose the music they preferred, and which was simpler to operate than existing apparatus already on the market. Such a device is now under development, and user feedback is being sought at each stage.

One of the more contentious areas of technology use is that of electronic tagging; that is, attaching some sort of device (a bracelet or a mobile phone) to the person with dementia, to enable them to be located. Miskelly (2004, 2005) examined the use of electronic tagging to address issues of 'wandering'[1] by people with dementia. The research found that devices in use for tagging prisoners as well as mobile phone technologies were effective in locating people with dementia who had gone out without a carer's knowledge. Miskelly (2004, p.306) notes that objections to tagging were raised by professional organizations, but not by people using services, their relatives or front-line staff. He argues that the electronic tagging approach was more acceptable and workable than physical or chemical restraint which might otherwise have been used in these cases. His work supports arguments about the need to look at technology in context, and to recognize that although technology might have originated in a negative context – monitoring prisoners – it can also be adapted to other contexts where it is considered important to know someone's whereabouts. This illustrates Baldwin's (2006) arguments about the values associated with technological devices. Here the fundamental value concerns a need to know where people are, and this may be for various purposes.

A particularly sensitive and careful use of electronic tracking using mobile phone technology has been reported from Paderborn in Germany (Körting 2005). The project began following the tragic death of a person with Alzheimer's disease who had become lost, and had not been located until 17 days later, when they had died of cold. Professionals from various disciplines met together to discuss how to prevent another such tragedy, and concluded that tracking using the global positioning system (GPS) would be useful. Technology was used in conjunction with careful individual assessments of each person's usual patterns of behaviour, and there was wide consultation with all those involved in each case, as well as a campaign to increase public awareness of dementia, and the possibilities of people becoming lost. This work is especially impressive for the way in which careful use of technology was employed to tackle a genuine issue, and for the ways in which many stakeholders were drawn together in the 'round table' which developed the scheme.

Lifestyle monitoring is a possible application of new technology whose use is little reported in the social care field. Fisk (2001,

---

1   Marshall (2001, p.127) notes that 'wandering' is 'a very misleading term for an activity that is usually purposeful, even if the purpose is not clear to those observing it'.

pp.217–220) outlines an evaluation of the use of lifestyle monitoring during 2000, known as the British Telecom/Anchor Trust initiative. This project involved using passive infrared (PIR) detectors throughout people's houses to record patterns of movement. Aberrant or uncharacteristic patterns for the individual concerned would raise alarms, which prompted a check with the resident to see whether all was well, followed by, as necessary, a call to an appropriate source of help. A difficulty arose concerning the identification of uncharacteristic behaviour, meaning that when the system should raise an alarm was difficult to determine. The users of the system were fairly positive about it, but they were very much a selected group, who had been persuaded to use the technology. Furthermore, many users were concerned about a feeling of being watched, the possible loss of contact with human sources of support and a feeling that the system might be used to save money rather than improve services. Fisk (2001) is critical of what he describes as the 'eulogistic' conclusions of the evaluation, as the reservations expressed even by enthusiastic clients were significant.

Technology in context

Other research has moved away from the focus on particular devices and has looked at the implementation of telecare in the context of local systems of care and support for older people, often linked to developments in smart housing.[2] Many of the projects evaluated have been small and temporary – Brownsell and Bradley (2003, pp.13–15), Fisk (2003, pp.189–193) and Woolham (2006b) list a number of examples – and few have focused specifically on people with dementia, or taken particular account of their needs.

Woolham's (2006a) evaluation of the 'Safe at Home' project in Northamptonshire was carried out between 2002 and 2004, following pilot work in 2001. It was a longitudinal study involving 233 people with a confirmed diagnosis of dementia who received items of technology to

---

2   'A smart home is one where smart technologies are installed and where those technologies facilitate automatic or user-initiated communication involving a range of appliances, sensors, actuators and switches' (Fisk 2003, p.179).

support them at home. Their outcomes, in terms of admissions to hospital or residential care, were compared with those of a group of similar people with dementia in another authority who did not receive technology. Costs of services were compared between the two authorities. Key questions for the study concerned the reliability of the technology, the extent to which it supported service users and informal carers, whether it promoted the maintenance of independence for users and its cost effectiveness. In this project, a wide range of technological items were used, with the large majority being 'stand-alone' types of equipment, and the most usual items being calendar clocks and medicine dispensers.

The evaluation found that effective use of technology required sensitive and responsive assessment systems, which could support good decisions about whether technology could be helpful, and, importantly, permit responses to changing needs. In particular, Woolham (2006a) notes the need to ensure that technology is in fact the correct solution for someone – an alternative might be a change in care practice. The study suggests that the attractions of technological devices and their promise of a quick and easy 'fix' may lead care managers to fail to consider other kinds of support, or underlying issues that may be masked. For informal carers, the study found that the technology could reduce stress, though it was important that technology provision was effectively tailored to people's particular needs, taking into account the varying ways in which people respond to the problems posed by dementia. For example, some carers were content for the person for whom they cared to be with them all the time, whilst others needed breaks. For people who needed breaks, the passive alarms were especially useful, as they could leave the person they cared for knowing that they could be called if help should be needed. Importantly, the study showed no reduction in human contact associated with the technology, and in many cases, improvements in self-esteem, dignity, quality of life and independence. The study demonstrated that the technology had produced significant cost savings, in terms of reduced admissions to hospitals and residential care, and had also reduced the costs of care at home.

The Northamptonshire study is important for demonstrating that technology really can improve quality of life for people with dementia and their carers. For care providers, the demonstration of cost savings is of particular interest, though the need for careful assessment and delivery of technological supports must also be carefully noted.

Another important evaluation is that of the West Lothian programme of smart technology and community care (Bowes and McColgan 2006). The West Lothian programme is not specific to people with dementia, but includes them in a radical new system of care and support for older people in general. The evaluation of the West Lothian programme was carried out between 2001 and 2005. In West Lothian, the local council took a decision in 1999 to overhaul its provision of care and support for older people radically. Faced with rising numbers of older people, several sub-standard care homes and a policy environment promoting community care for older people, the Council decided to use smart technology both in people's own, existing homes in the community and in newly built housing complexes which would offer housing with care.

Following assessment of needs, all clients would have a basic technology package in their home. This would consist of a home alert console connected to a call centre and a basic set of alarm devices, namely two passive infrared (PIR) detectors which could detect movement or lack of it; two flood detectors; one heat extreme sensor, which could identify both heat and cold; and one smoke detector. These devices could be augmented with many other pieces of technology, assessed as being appropriate for the individual concerned. Alarms were either passive (such as the smoke alarm in the basic package) or active (such as pendant alarms, given to all existing community alarm clients). Other equipment included door entry systems or remote control devices for doors, windows, curtains and so on. The call centre had individually tailored protocols for every client, with appropriate courses of action, such as phoning the client to check how things were, calling a relative or calling a support or emergency service, depending on the nature of the alarm raised. New staff teams were built to provide support in the community and in the housing with care developments, with staff from a range of backgrounds, including residential care, occupational therapy, housing work and nursing.

The evaluation involved exploring in depth the views and experiences of 81 service users and informal carers and 77 staff, a detailed costs analysis involving over 100 individual cases and a review of a comparator group of older people from another, similar authority. By the latter stages of the evaluation, more than 2000 technology packages had been installed.

People who had received technology packages installed in the community felt that they were being supported to remain in their own homes, which were their preferred residences. The technology meant that they knew help would come if they were in difficulties, and they appreciated the regular checks with the call centre. Many people had informal carers who were very important to them, and who, in turn, felt that the technology gave them increased peace of mind, and reduced their caring burdens, improving their relationships with the person for whom they cared. Staying in one's own home could permit the maintenance of good neighbourly relationships, and, where people lived in less desirable neighbourhoods, the technology helped to maintain security at home.

In the new developments, clients and informal carers reported improvements in their feelings of safety and security. Clients felt that, although they had moved home, the flats and cottages to which they had moved still felt like home, and supported independent living. Informal carers reported less stress. As the new developments were based locally, tenants maintained their local networks and, as time went on, new community relationships were built within the developments themselves.

For staff, the innovations produced changes in culture, from an emphasis on care to one of support and capacity building. The new teams were unfamiliar at first, but staff explained that these had helped them to review their ways of working and to develop a new approach to their work – this was especially the case for the front-line staff in the support teams, and the impact on care managers was less marked.

The evaluation revealed a number of specific issues for people with dementia. First, there was an effort to 'mainstream' them into the system which was intended to be available to all, and to adapt to people's changing needs, involving changes in physical and/or cognitive capacity. This is in tune with an approach to work with people with dementia which emphasizes personhood and inclusivity in models of care. Second, in the early stages of the programme, technology packages were allocated to people who were 'at risk' of going into hospital or residential care, often as a result of a crisis situation. It became clear rapidly that, especially for people with dementia, the technology packages could not make a difference at this stage. Decisions were taken therefore to install technology at a much earlier point, and the later stages of the evaluation suggested that this was more effective. Third, there were issues attached to stereotypes of people with dementia which focused on incapacity. There was evidence that some care managers and front-line staff did not see potential for technology packages to support people with dementia, especially as the disease progressed. During the course of the programme, it proved necessary to check that people with dementia were indeed being recommended for packages, rather than assumed incapable of benefiting from them – the evaluation found that people with dementia were being included, despite resistance among some staff, and that the managers were conscious of the need for vigilance in this respect.

The West Lothian case is important because it is almost certainly the largest implementation of telecare in the world, in terms of the number of clients and the length of time the system has been in operation. The evaluation suggests that the model of care in West Lothian has delivered benefits for clients in terms of greater independence and better quality of life and for informal carers in terms of peace of mind and much needed support. The Council also derived benefits in terms of cost effective services, which support the meeting of targets, such as reducing the numbers of long-stay hospital beds, in which West Lothian has been outstandingly successful. Despite the issues identified and the continuing efforts to improve in this area, the benefits include support for people with dementia. One of the most significant elements of the system is the focus on mainstreaming, which became increasingly important in the later stages of the evaluation with a decision to extend availability of the basic package to everyone in West Lothian aged 60 and over who wished to have it in their homes, regardless of need for services. This element of the programme was aimed at removing stigma attached to receipt of services, in that the basic system would become an ordinary part of people's lives, which might or might not be modified as their needs for care and support changed.

Issues in evaluating technology for dementia care

Ethical issues

Ethics have been an important topic of debate in relation to the use of technology in dementia care. Pioneering work carried out by the ASTRID
project (Marshall 2000) is especially important in these debates, and sets
out a benchmark for ethical review in the area. The work of the ASTRID
project was founded on the principle that the primary concern must be the
views and wishes of the person with dementia themselves, and the
improvement of their quality of life (Marshall 2000, p.12). The ASTRID
guide adopts an approach to ethics first set out by Hope and Oppenheimer
(1997), known as the 'three Ps' – perspectives, principles and paradigms.
These highlight matters to be considered when examining the ethics of
using technology in dementia care. As Marshall (2000) points out, matters
are not necessarily simple, and ethical questions have to be considered on a
case-by-case basis. In all cases, however, the *perspectives* of those involved in
receiving the service must be considered, and their views about providing
or not providing the technology sought. The *principles* which must be
applied are conventional to ethical practice generally and involve respect
for the person concerned, beneficence, non-maleficence and justice. The
reference to *paradigms* suggests the comparison of cases with others – for
example, considering whether a decision being made in the case of a
person with dementia is similar to one which would be made in the case of
someone with learning disabilities. Such comparison can help identify
whether the person with dementia is being treated justly, with respect for
their personhood. It should be noted that some of the technology is particularly powerful, necessitating scrupulous attention to ethical issues.

The research discussed earlier has paid significant attention to ethical
issues throughout. Ethical committees have been consulted for approval,
sometimes presenting difficulties for researchers working with very new
devices (for example, Jones 2005) in addition to the difficulties of involving people with dementia in research. Any evaluation will face ethical
issues, and it is important that continuing discussion takes place on these.
In particular, it is important, in a rapidly developing field such as the use of
technology, that emerging issues are identified and addressed, rather than,
as has been the case in the past, a focus on a rather narrowly defined and

predetermined set of issues (Baldwin *et al.* 2003). For example, Hughes *et al.* (2002a, 2002b) identify issues of ethics faced by informal carers, which are related to often complex relationships with those for whom they care. They highlight the case of an intimate partner having to progressively deprive the person for whom they care of former freedoms, such as use of the car, choice of attire and, perhaps, freedom itself.

User perspectives

Barron *et al.* (2004), whose focus is predominantly medical research, suggest that some formal ethical procedures have made it more difficult for researchers to involve people with dementia in research. They argue for a balance to be struck between protecting people with dementia, and ensuring that the research is done, in accordance with the work cited here.

User perspectives are important at the design stage, through the development of products, to the establishment and delivery of services. Crabtree *et al.* (2003) argue that good design and, it can be added, good quality services adapt to the 'lives and rhythms' of older people. Certainly, one of the main findings of research on older people's views about services in general is that they prefer those which tune into their preferred lifestyles and daily habits, rather than those which disrupt these (see Kellaher 2001).

There is now much research which demonstrates conclusively that the views of people with dementia can be ascertained, and that people with dementia are interested in and want to participate in decision making about the care and support services supplied for them. Researchers who have discussed this in detail and developed ways of ascertaining people's views include Wilkinson (2001) and Hubbard *et al.* (2002). The views of people with dementia about technology have not been widely reported, as we have noted above, but there are clear precedents demonstrating both the possibility and the desirability of including them. Their views can be relevant both at the stage of the development of products and also once services are rolled out. The positive impact of user consultation on the effectiveness and acceptability of services has been widely reported in other fields of care for older people (see Andrews, Manthorpe and Watson

2004) and there is every reason to expect positive results from older people with dementia using technology.

In the light of such research and the innovative methods of consultation and data collection developed in recent years, it is somewhat surprising that so much technological development is technology rather than user driven. Nevertheless, Sixsmith (2006) has noted that this is still the case, and that service development has to challenge this perspective.

It is also important to challenge wider ageist stereotypes which suggest that older people may not be able to cope with technological innovation. Certainly in the Northampton and West Lothian evaluations discussed earlier, older people, including people with dementia and family carers (often spouses of similar age), were able and willing to express their views about technology, at all stages of the processes of assessment, installation and use. These findings support those of a significant body of research, cited by Fisk (2001, pp.117–119), demonstrating that older people are both keen and critical users of new technologies. Marshall's (2001, p.138) case study of 'Mrs McFee' who disliked a technology installation so much that she threw it out of the front door is a reminder of the strong ways in which a person with dementia may make their views known.

Models of care

The research record to date emphasizes the importance of understanding the context in which technologies are deployed. Devices can be used (and potentially misused) in a variety of care models. As Fisk (2003) makes clear, the history of community alarms is varied, and they have been used in a range of different ways. If smart technologies represent continuity with older community alarm systems, we should naturally expect that they too will vary in their implementation. The very different approaches taken by Northamptonshire, with the emphasis on stand-alone devices, and West Lothian, with the authority-wide commitment to smart technology linked to a call centre, are cases in point.

The West Lothian model of care is one which innovates in terms of breaking down the boundaries between different professional disciplines. Whilst this was challenging for staff, the researchers suggested that the technology itself, being so new to most of the staff involved, aided in the process of developing new work teams and new care practices (Bowes and McColgan 2006). Technology in this case worked as a catalyst for change, a point also noted by Barlow (2005). Whilst the West Lothian approach produced mainly positive outcomes, in other cases organizational imperatives may not necessarily benefit service users – May *et al.* (2003) cite a number of examples of the use of telemedicine in which the organizational imperative to cut costs did not improve patient care.

Costs

Considerations of costs have been an important driver for innovations in the use of new technologies. With the population of older people set to increase significantly in coming decades, the issue of the costs of long-term care has come to the fore. Since the increasing numbers are particularly marked for the older age groups, increases are projected in the numbers of people with dementia. Thus evidence that the use of technology in dementia care can cut costs has been eagerly sought. Existing research has started to indicate that there may well be cost savings, as we have noted above. Outcome measures in costing work in this area have focused particularly on the extent to which people receiving technological support have remained in their own homes, rather than moving to hospital or residential care. The Northampton study has shown particular benefits in this regard. However, available statistics on community care outcomes tend to be poor, as record keeping and management systems in local authorities in the UK are not necessarily set up for ready access for monitoring and research purposes – Barlow (2005) makes a plea for improvements in this area, and for the ready accessibility of data to allow comparisons between systems. The potentiality of technological systems to collect data about themselves – such as frequency of calls – can be advantageous here, though such facilities require considered use.

There are particular difficulties in relation to accurate data about people with dementia, because only people with a formal diagnosis can be identified as representing a larger population of people who may have significant cognitive impairment, but have not sought a diagnosis. Data for the general population of older people are therefore significant for people with dementia, as many will be included.

Magnusson and Hanson (2003), however, caution against too strong an emphasis on costs in their review of ethical issues in supplying information and communication technology to older people and family carers. They feel that the key questions are of quality of life and enhancing care and support for older people. Nevertheless, as Brownsell and Bradley (2003, p.50) point out, telecare will not be widely used unless its costs and benefits are well understood. Their analysis suggests that there is considerable potential for savings, as noted above.

Staffing issues

One rather neglected area of research has been the impact of new technologies for staff involved in caring for people with dementia. We have already noted how new technologies can challenge staff in their customary practice, and how, if they are introduced at system level, they may imply wholesale change. There are implications for implementing technology-based changes, such as a need for staff training, not least in the ethical issues attached to using technology. Magnusson and Hanson (2003) add that staff need to be convinced of the benefits of a technological intervention, or they may prevent its use to its full potential. Holland and Peace (2001) see moves towards more integrated services, which many systems of smart technology certainly involve, as presenting challenges for staff teams and organizations alike, and suggest that these should be expected as part of the process of integration.

Conclusion

Research so far therefore suggests that new technologies, both as separate items and as part of telecare systems, can be of significant benefit for people with dementia, their carers and those who supply services to them. In this rapidly changing field, however, there is a continuing need for what Barlow (2005) refers to as 'pragmatic evaluation', which recognizes the complexity and variety of systems in use, whilst collecting systematic data about their impact and effectiveness. Technology is undoubtedly powerful, potentially risky and could be used in unethical ways. Learning from good practice, being aware of potential problems, reflecting on local practice and realizing the potential of new technologies to enhance quality of life (see Fisk 2001; Marshall 2001) can all be supported by effective dissemination of research results, and the accessibility of reports, many of which are currently difficult to find. In this regard, the Department of Health's website at www.icesdoh.org/doc_cat.asp?ID=6 which contains many documents and reports about telecare and advice on implementation is to be welcomed.

Any pragmatic evaluation needs to address ethical issues, as suggested, and these are likely to shift with technological development. This is an area in which communication is particularly important. The significance of user views has already been established, and their incorporation into evaluation is now part of good practice as well as a policy imperative. Pragmatic evaluation of necessity entails understanding the model of care within which technology is being used. The concern with costs is inevitable, and research to date suggests that benefits for both providers and users can accrue from technology, well used. Staffing issues have been somewhat neglected, but are central to successful implementation.

Some of the greatest enthusiasm for technology therefore perhaps requires to be tempered, in that it provides a set of tools, rather than a fully developed approach to supporting people with dementia. The issue for care providers is to learn from and build on existing experience to use technology in the most effective ways.

References

Andrews, J.A., Manthorpe, J. and Watson, R. (2004) 'Involving older people in intermediate care.' *Journal of Advanced Nursing 46*, 3, 303–310.

Baldwin, C. (2006) 'Reflections on ethics, dementia and technology.' In J. Woolham (ed.) *Assistive Technology in Dementia Care. Developing the Role of Technology in the Care and Rehabilitation of People with Dementia – Current Trends and Perspectives.* London: Hawker Publications. pp.54–66.

Baldwin, C., Hughes, J., Hope, T., Jacoby, R. and Ziebland, S. (2003) 'Ethics and dementia: mapping the literature by bibliometric analysis.' *International Journal of Geriatric Psychiatry 18*, 1, 41–54.

Barlow, J. (2005) *Building an Evidence Base for Successful Telecare Implementation – Report of the Evidence Working Group of the Telecare Policy Collaborative.* www.icesdoh.org/downloads/Factsheet%20-%20Telecare%20-%20Evidence%20-%208%20August%202005.doc. Consulted January 2006.

Barron, J.S., Duffey, P.L., Byrd, L.J., Campbell, R. and Ferrucci, L. (2004) 'Informed consent for research participation in frail older persons.' *Aging Clinical and Experimental Research 16*, 1, 79–85.

Bowes, A.M. and McColgan, G.M. (2006) *Smart Technology and Community Care for Older People.* Edinburgh: Age Concern Scotland.

Brownsell, S. and Bradley, D. (2003) *Assistive Technology and Telecare: Forging Solutions for Independent Living.* Bristol: Policy Press.

Crabtree, A., Hemmings, T., Rodden, T., Cheverst, K., Clarke, K., Dewsbury, G., Hughes, J. and Rouncefield, M. (2003) 'Designing with care: adapting cultural probes to inform design in sensitive settings.' In *Proceedings of OzCHI 2003, New Directions in Interaction: Information Environments, Media and Technology*, 26–28 November at the University of Queensland, Brisbane, Australia. pp.4–13.

Department of Health (2005) *Building Telecare in England.* www.dh.gov.uk/PolicyAndGuidance/HealthAndSocialCareTopics/OlderPeoplesServices/OlderPeopleArticle/fs/en?CONTENT_ID=4116208&chk=g6m5JL. Consulted January 2006.

ENABLE (2005) Project website. www.enableproject.org/. Consulted January 2006.

Fisk, M.J. (2001) 'The implications of smart home technologies.' In S.M. Peace and C. Holland (eds) *Inclusive Design in an Ageing Society: Innovative Approaches.* Bristol: Policy Press. pp.101–124.

Fisk, M.J. (2003) *Social Alarms to Telecare: Older People's Services in Transition.* Bristol: Policy Press.

Hagen, I., Holthe, T., Gilliard, J., Topo, P., Cahill, S., Begley, E., Jones, K., Duff, P., Macijauskiene, J., Budraitiene, A., Bjørneby, S. and Engedal, K. (2004) 'Development of a protocol for the assessment of assistive aids for people with dementia.' *Dementia 3*, 3, 281–296.

Holland, C. and Peace, S.M. (2001) 'Inclusive housing.' In S.M. Peace and C. Holland (eds) *Inclusive Design in an Ageing Society: Innovative Approaches.* Bristol: Policy Press. pp.235–260.

Hope, T. and Oppenheimer, C. (1997) 'Ethics and the psychiatry of old age.' In R. Jacoby and C. Oppenheimer (eds) *Psychiatry in the Elderly.* Oxford: Oxford University Press. pp.709–735.

Hubbard, G., Cook, A., Tester, S. and Downs, C. (2002) 'Beyond words: older people with dementia using and interpreting non-verbal behaviour.' *Journal of Aging Studies 16*, 2, 155–167.

Hughes, J.C., Hope, T., Reader, S. and Rice, D. (2002a) 'Dementia and ethics: the views of informal carers.' *Journal of the Royal Society of Medicine 95*, 5, 242–246.

Hughes, J.C., Hope, T., Savulescu, J. and Ziebland, S. (2002b) 'Carers, ethics and dementia: a survey and review of the literature.' *International Journal of Geriatric Psychiatry 17*, 1, 35–40.

Jones, K. (2005) *Enabling Technologies for People with Dementia (ENABLE): Report of the Assessment Study in England.* www.enableproject.org/download/Enable%20-%20National%20Report%20-%20UK.pdf. Consulted January 2006.

Kellaher, L. (2001) 'Shaping everyday life: beyond design.' In S.M. Peace and C. Holland (eds) *Inclusive Housing in an Ageing Society: Innovative Approaches.* Bristol: Policy Press. pp.215–234.

Körting, S. (2005) *Projekt 'Suche nach verwirrten Menschen' – das Paderborn Modell*. (Project 'Looking for confused people' – the Paderborn Model) www.alzheimer-paderborn. de/index-Dateien/Projektbericht_Suche_nach_verwirrten_Menschen.pdf. Consulted January 2006.

Magnusson, L. and Hanson, E.J. (2003) 'Ethical issues arising from a research, technology and development project to support frail older people and their family carers at home.' *Health and Social Care in the Community 11*, 5, 431–439.

Manthorpe, J. (2004) 'Risk taking.' In A. Innes, C. Archibald and C. Murphy (eds) *Dementia and Social Inclusion: Marginalised Groups and Marginalised Areas of Dementia Research, Care and Practice*. London: Jessica Kingsley Publishers. pp.137–149.

Marshall, M. (2000) *ASTRID: A Social and Technological Response to Meeting the Needs of Individuals with Dementia and their Carers*. London: Hawker Publications.

Marshall, M. (2001) 'Dementia and technology.' In S.M. Peace and C. Holland (eds) *Inclusive Design in an Ageing Society: Innovative Approaches*. Bristol: Policy Press. pp.125–143.

May, C.R. (2005) *Telemedicine and the 'Future Patient'? Risk, Governance and Innovation: Final Report to ESRC*. Project ref: L21825 2067. www.regard.ac.uk/ESRCInfoCentre/ index.aspx. Consulted January 2006.

May, C., Mort, M., Williams, T., Mair, F. and Gask, L. (2003) 'Health technology assessment in its local contexts: studies of telehealthcare.' *Social Science and Medicine 57*, 5, 697–710.

Miskelly, F. (2004) 'A novel system of electronic tagging in patients with dementia and wandering.' *Age and Ageing 33*, 3, 304–306.

Miskelly, F. (2005) 'Electronic tracking of patients with dementia and wandering using mobile phone technology.' *Age and Ageing 34*, 5, 497–499.

Sixsmith, A. (2006) 'New technologies to support independent living and quality of life for people with dementia.' *Alzheimer's Care Quarterly* (in press).

Sixsmith, A. and Gibson, G. (2006) 'Music and the well-being of people with dementia.' *Ageing and Society 26* (in press).

Topo, P. and Saarikalle, K. (2005) *Enabling Technologies for People with Dementia (ENABLE): Report of Picture Gramophone Assessment: National Results from Finland, Ireland, Norway and UK and Cross National Results*. www.enableproject.org/download/Enable%20-%20 Report%20-%20PG%20hybrid10.5.pdf. Consulted January 2006.

Topo, P., Saarikalle, K., Mäki, O. and Parviainen, S. (2005) *Enabling Technologies for People with Dementia (ENABLE): Report of Assessment Study in Finland*. www.enable project.org/download/Enable%20-%20National%20Report%20-%20Finland.pdf. Consulted January 2006.

Wilkinson, H. (ed.) (2001) *The Perspectives of People with Dementia: Research Methods and Motivations*. London: Jessica Kingsley Publishers.

Woolham, J. (2006a) *Safe at Home – The Effectiveness of Assistive Technology in Supporting the Independence of People with Dementia: The Safe at Home Project*. London: Hawker Publications.

Woolham, J. (2006b) *Assistive Technology in Dementia Care. Developing the Role of Technology in the Care and Rehabilitation of People with Dementia – Current Trends and Perspectives*. London: Hawker Publications.

Chapter 6

Evaluating Long Stay Care Settings
The Environment

Helle Wijk

An increasing number of research and evaluative studies focus on the physical aspects of the environment as an important dimension of caring for people with dementia and their quality of life, with the assumption that some of this control may be built into the way the nursing home is designed (Lawton 2001; Mozley, Huxley and Cordingly 1999). Environmental factors may have both a supportive and a hindering effect on adequate performance, interaction with family, fellow-residents and staff, and an individual's feelings of security and safety (Day, Carreon and Stump 2000). Adapting the environment with the intention of matching it to the needs of the user may be considered a non-pharmacological treatment, as environmental factors can be easier to alter than pathological factors influencing the situation of the person with dementia (Zeisel 2000). In several studies interaction and prevalence of adequate performance have been designated as measures of the success of an environmental intervention. Better knowledge about the interaction between people with dementia and their living environment, and the importance of the environment, can be crucial for planning, designing and evaluating the caring environments for people with dementia.

This chapter begins by describing the ecological model of ageing which highlights the impact of the environment for older people and people with dementia. The links between ageing and the environment are explored using this model and specific aspects of the environment including colour and sound are examined in more detail. A discussion follows on how the impact of design features can be evaluated and the chapter concludes with future directions in this area.

The need for special care units in old age and in dementia

There is a need for special care units (SCU) for people with dementia, designed according to the needs of those living there and staffed with competent and motivated employees (Cohen and Day 1993; Kelly 1993). SCUs should promote physiological support, safety, belonging, self-esteem and self-expression by focusing on the physical environment together with therapeutic programmes and the involvement of staff and relatives (Berg *et al.* 1991) According to Lawton (2001) there are four general user-related aims of environmental interventions: *decreasing disturbing behaviour, increasing social behaviour, increasing activity* and *increasing positive feelings and decreasing negative feelings.* Liebowitz, Lawton and Waldman (1979) were able to demonstrate increased social activities and interest in the physical surroundings as a result of interventions such as colour coding the bedrooms and using bright colours to attract patients' attention at an institution for confused people. Küller (1991) described similar effects as a result of a more home-like design at an institution for individuals with dementia and the importance of an easy floor plan configuration together with concrete signs and symbols has also been highlighted (Passini *et al.* 1998). Avoiding glare and the use of pastel colours and more frequent use of contrasting colours to facilitate orientation and functioning have been suggested to be important (Cannava 1994). Passini *et al.* (2000) reported a way-finding experience performed with individuals suffering from advanced Alzheimer's disease in which even people with severe cognitive decline were able to reach certain destinations. The availability of readily accessible environmental information, a great number of reference points and the avoidance of floor patterns and dark lines that could increase anxiety were all found to be critical features in the environment.

Adapting the environment to special needs in old age

To take an interest in *preserved* environmental perception in old age instead
of its *losses* is in a way to reconsider caring for older people, moving away
from a focus on risk factors for pathology and towards a focus on health-
promoting issues instead. This approach, also called the salutogenic way of
caring (Antonovsky 1987), advocates that the focus of caring should be on
individuals' residual health rather than disease. In connection with that,
Antonovsky (1987) emphasized that caring should take into account what
other measures beside medical care could promote health for the person.
This focus on health and preserved functions rather than disease and lost
functions is also in line with the concept of patient empowerment, defined
as giving the individual the opportunity to engage in and influence his or
her care and rehabilitation (Baksi and Cradock 1998). By focusing on preserved function, and by implementing this knowledge in the environment
and care of the old, the aim is to foster opportunities for patients to behave
independently. This is congruent with the central concept of nursing
science: person, environment, health and nursing. The characteristic
features of nursing are the respect and dignity for the person as a whole in
his or her environment with the overall goal of contributing to health and
supporting preserved functions. This is expressed in many nursing
theories, for example Orem's (1995) model of nursing with its focus on
compensation for the patient's lack of self-care abilities. Based on the
knowledge of how the older person with dementia perceives the environment the nurse could contribute to an enhanced visibility and understanding of the environment in many ways. For example, more frequent use of
contrasts, cues and codes could increase the possibilities of independent
functioning and decrease the barriers to it (Wijk in progress).

The increase in research stressing the importance of environmental
design on the quality of life for older persons (Kayser-Jones 1991; Lawton
2001) complements the fact that competent cognitive functioning, that is
the ability to perform activities in everyday living and engaging in the
meaningful use of time and social behaviour, has been shown to be of
equal importance to persons with dementia as to the population at large
(Lawton 1994). Only a few years ago systematic guidelines for providing
optimal environmental input to meet the needs of the persons with

dementia were more or less absent. Today there is a fast growing body of evidence-based design suggestions informing the design of residential environments for people with dementia. But even though the knowledge base comprises a variety of methods, regrettably few can serve as hard facts or design directives.

There are of course many factors influencing how we perceive and are able to function in the environment. The feeling of safety, for instance, is a major concern when designing environments for older people, and achieving it has been shown to be a very complicated task. Aspects such as type of walking surface, visual aspects and ambient conditions must interact with those aspects of ageing which involve visual and auditory perception, balance, orientation and cognition.

There are several approaches to understanding how institutional environments affect adaptation in old age. Summarizing these, the concept of environmental pressure is used to predict outcomes in individual cases with salient individual characteristics in the conceptual models including coping, competence and personality traits.

The ecological model of ageing

The characteristic feature of the ecological model of ageing, developed by Lawton and Nahemow (1973), is that it predicts behavioural outcomes by looking at an individual's competence in relation to environmental pressure. The model is built on the equation $B = f(P, E)$, where B stands for behaviour and is conceptualized as a function, f, of the combination of P, the person or competence, and E, the environment.

Competence is only a part of the person (P) which includes a person's biological health, sensory perceptual capacity, motor skills, cognitive capacity and ego strength. Adaptation is predicted by examining the match between competence and the demands of the environment. Environmental pressure (E) encompasses the multiple demands of the environment upon the individual. It includes aspects of the physical environment (lighting, orientation cues, geographic distance), the personal environment (family members, friends and so on), the supra-personal environment (characteristics of the residents in a person's neighbourhood), and the social environment (norms, values in the individual's society).

According to the model the environments are classified on the basis of the 'demand character' of the context in which the person acts. The demand character could be positive, neutral or negative. When the capacity of the individual is in balance with the pressure of the environment the demand character is neutral. If the individual competence deteriorates, the pressure from the environment must decrease as well in order to remain in balance. Outcomes for individuals are dependent upon the strength of environmental pressure in relation to an individual's adaptation level and his or her competence. The less competent the individual is, the greater the impact of environmental factors on that individual (Lawton and Nahemow 1973). The outcome, when a person of a given level of competence is acting in an environment with a given pressure level, could be placed on a continuum from positive to negative and is manifested on two levels, as behaviour and affect. Thereby it would be possible to predict behavioural outcomes by looking at an individual's competence in relation to environmental pressure.

Nursing is sometimes described as the sum of knowledge from many disciplines synthesized into caring for the entire human being. The common goals of taking charge of preserved functions to promote health, support independence and always taking individuals' whole competences into consideration is essential in caring. There have been several studies using the ecological model as a framework for nursing actions in adapting the environment to the needs of older people and people with dementia. Sandman (1986) found that observed improvements in Activities of Daily Living (ADL) functions after relocation to a more positive environment for people with dementia could be related to the model. Environments better adapted to individuals' competences could lead to increases in those individuals' inherent capacities. A similar conclusion was reached in relation to increasing function in meal behaviour among patients with dementia after adaptation of the environment to meet the patients' capacity (Sandman 1986). Gustavsson (1996) takes another approach when referring to the model by modifying the activities instead of the environment. Her study concerns quality of life and functional capacity during locomotor disability. She points out that the patients were at high risk of being hindered in behaviour by their disability but with alterations to activities the environmental pressure could be changed from negative to positive.

Reduction of environmental pressure by modification of the environment

Reducing environmental pressure to meet the normal sensory and physiological changes that occur with ageing and dementia has been the focus of multi-disciplinary interest by both researchers and practitioners within gerontology over the years (Cannava 1994; Kayser-Jones 1991; Lawton 1994; Pastalan 1997). The impact of the environment on health and well-being is also one of the hallmarks of many nursing theories (for example, Nightingale 1969; Watson 1985).

The ageing process itself and specific dementia-related processes affect the level of individual competence, and most likely also the ability to handle the environmental pressure. Although studies of older people indicate that a majority of older people remain in good physical and mental condition over time, it is still a fact that chronic disease and disability become more frequent with increasing age (Heikkinen *et al.* 1997). Common changes, for example in sensory acuity, psychomotor speed, mobility, social roles and cognitive function, make older people more reliant on the physical environment. The combined effects of these changes could be summarized as difficulties in acquiring and retaining spatially-bound information and recognizing features.

However, even though older age is related to an increasing risk of cognitive decline and visual disturbance, it does not necessarily mean a negative change in performance. On the contrary, it has been shown that personality factors and the ability to use different coping strategies to overcome difficulties in daily life and to maintain a high degree of activity level are the major determinants of well-being among the oldest old (Hillerås 2000). It has also been assumed that supportive environmental layouts could have positive impacts on the behaviour of individuals despite loss of functions (Lawton 1994). In addition, factors such as activity, lifestyle, social network and the living environment have been suggested as important to the capacity to survive as opposed to chronological age itself. Emphasizing preserved functions, improvement in the environment and patient–staff interaction have been shown to reduce patients' dependency to some extent and to improve function (Sandman 1986). Studies within the architectural field focusing on the demands that a health-promoting, patient-focused perspective puts on the planning and design of hospitals provide another expression of these findings (Dunlop 1993).

It is essential that the whole team working with the patient is aware of the impact of the environment upon the quality of care for older people. By doing so they may be instrumental in reducing some of the harmful effects of poor environmental design. The focus is on how to maximize the use of older people's capacities in the environment with the aim of finding means to compensate for normal and pathological specific loss of function in individuals. For example, collaboration between architecture and nursing could be expanded when planning for new institutions so as to promote a better understanding of the special needs of these residents. Evaluation of the individual's personal competence should lead to different approaches in order to adapt the environmental pressure and promote independent functioning.

Colour in the environment

Colour is of great importance for most people in most environments for the detection and identification of objects, for information purposes, and from an aesthetic point of view. Normally perceptual information of the environment is sufficient, but the visual and cognitive deterioration that accompany ageing can have a negative impact on how we perceive and act in the environment. Karatza (1995) offers guidelines on how to use colours in the environment of older people based on research and experiments with older people compared to younger control groups. In her work she emphasizes, for example, the importance of using colour contrasts to increase visibility, of colour coding and cueing to support object identification, and of a conscious colour scheme to make the environment attractive. These recommendations, however, do not take people with dementia specifically into consideration.

Cooper (1999) has conducted several intervention studies over the years, trying to measure the effect of conscious use of colour in the environment for older people. These interventions were able to show that neutral colours and lack of contrast minimize attention when compared to strong colour cues, which seem to attract attention. The former, therefore, may be used as a way to prevent behaviour such as walking into restricted areas; the latter may be used to improve the visual distinction of objects.

Wijk's studies (Wijk 1998, 2001; Wijk and Sivik 1995; Wijk *et al.* 1999a, 1999b, 2001, 2002) of environmental interventions for older people with declining visual and cognitive functions indicate, in line with the ecological model of ageing (Lawton and Nahemow 1973), the possibilities for preventing differences between older people's levels of adaptation and the demands posed by their surroundings. More frequent use of contrasting colours is proposed in order to accomplish visual distinction in the environment, to support depth and spatial perception and to simplify object recognition. Colours similar in lightness could be juxtaposed when the purpose is to camouflage and minimize attention. Shades of different lightness within the red and yellow coloured area on the walls of the room could support spatial distinction. Coding and cueing presuppose a communication between the carer and patient based upon a common understanding of the concept. Therefore, a more frequent use of the elementary colours (blue, red, green, yellow, black and white) for codes and cues in the environment could be recommended in contrast to some of the mixed colours causing problems for a majority of the participants (turquoise, pink, orange and purple). Because deteriorating vision is common with ageing, very dark or light colours should be avoided as codes and cues since they seem to be difficult to distinguish.

Colour preferences remain more or less stable throughout life and since colour and colour design are highly appreciated among older people it is appropriate that colour designs in environments for older people should take into account the colour preferences of the inhabitants. It is suggested that colour could be used to draw attention to cues in the environment of older people. The shape of cues and their associations seem to be more important in supporting recognition in the longer term. Therefore, in order to make older people aware of the cues they need to be communicated between carers and patients, and they need to be clearly visible in the environment.

Despite the evidence-based recommendations mentioned above (see Wijk 2001) there have not been many systematic attempts to evaluate the advantages of clear colour designs for older people and people with dementia. In a recent intervention study conducted at a nursing home for people with dementia in Sweden, it was possible to show important effects following the implementation of a complete new colour design at the nursing home that was intended to decrease stress and increase orientation and the feeling of security among the inhabitants. The study was the result of close collaboration between researchers, architects, the staff and management at the nursing home, the relatives of the inhabitants and the painters and decorators. At baseline the number of falls among the inhabitants in the previous six months and the work satisfaction of the staff were measured. Relatives of the residents were interviewed about their opinion of the quality of the physical environment.

After the baseline measures were completed an intensive intervention period began. This encompassed the overall colour scheme, the floor carpeting, the bathroom environment and the illumination of the nursing home. A light background colour was used for the corridors, hallways and entrances into the staff rest-rooms and offices, with the entrances into the residents' apartments, the dining room and the kitchen highlighted with a reddish marker around the doors. The floor carpet was changed throughout the nursing home, with a lighter colour devoid of contrast effects used between the rooms and corridor in order to avoid misinterpretation of floor levels. In the bathrooms a contrasting blue colour was used behind the white water basin and toilet to support perception and independence. The illumination all over the nursing home was improved using a high degree of general ceiling illumination complemented by plenty of individualized spotlights to support visibility when reading, eating, sewing and doing other activities. When, three months after the baseline measures, the intervention was finished, the same measures were repeated. The result showed a decrease in the number of falls, an increase in work satisfaction among the staff and increased levels of confidence in the residents from their relatives (Wijk in progress).

Illumination of the environment

Older people commonly have insufficient illumination in their homes, and this can have an unnecessarily negative effect on their quality of life (Brunnström *et al.* 2004). For older people still living at home the most important action is to change or complement the existing illumination with lighting of a better and more functional quality. Nursing homes often lack variation and flexibility when considering the illumination of communal rooms. In the dining room, illumination that both supports activities and provides a comfortable atmosphere is needed, and good lighting over the kitchen table focusing on the table and food supports independence during the meal (Bowers, Meek and Stewart 2001).

Sound in the environment

For people with dementia even slight changes in the environment can be hazardous and difficult to interpret. A calm ward atmosphere that promotes a relaxed environment in which sounds that are not recognized by the residents are avoided or camouflaged and good sounds that support recognition and joy are clearly audible should be encouraged. Mobile phones should be avoided, as should music that is not familiar to residents. An important intervention is to control for the needs of people with hearing aids. Playing soft background music during dinner can be a way to decrease anxiousness and agitation at a nursing home. The effect of music in the caring environment is frequently under-estimated, but it can be crucial as uncontrolled music can have negative effects. It is important to highlight the positive effects of music in the care of older people and people with dementia. It is well known that people with dementia who have severe language deficits can both handle musical instruments and sing along. Music activities can be both collective or individual and, even when residents cannot join the activity, the music can still affect the atmosphere in a positive way. Playing music at a nursing home can be a stimulating activity that evokes positive memories and joy in residents. Through music it may be possible to communicate with people who have lost their ability to communicate verbally. It can decrease agitation and worry and so have a positive effect on care. It has also been shown that music can have a pain-relieving effect, distracting the patient from the feeling of pain (Ragneskog 2001).

Evaluating the impact or usefulness of environmental factors

An overview of the increasing number of studies on design and dementia reveals a variety of methods for evaluating outcomes. One critical issue to take into consideration is the fact that dementia progresses during the intervention, resulting in possible influences on the structure, process and results of the intervention. In such circumstances it is difficult to know whether it is the effect of the redesign or the progress of the dementia that is being evaluated. This is a clear finding of the empirical research presented in the literature, within which both experimental and longitudinal studies are scarce. One reason could be, as highlighted by Lawton (2001), that many environmental assessment instruments comprise descriptive materials that do not fit easily into evaluative frameworks designed to determine how well environmental design elements perform in terms of meeting users' needs. Research strategies that may be used to evaluate the effect of environmental design in dementia care settings include consumer surveys, direct behaviour observation, expert judgements or experimental design and environmental trials.

The logic of using consumer surveys for evaluation is clearly to ask the experts, that is to say the residents with all their experience of living in different types of nursing homes, to assess the quality of care and the context of care. The main limitation of this method is the difficulties that people with dementia experience both in evaluating their environment and in sharing this information with others. Another limitation of this method is that most standard questionnaires are quite complex in nature with a lack of focus on environmental items. Improvements are being made in terms of ongoing attempts to construct specific questionnaires addressing the subjective quality of life within the range of possible responses for people with mild to moderate dementia (Lawton 2001).

Direct behaviour observations attempt to evaluate and relate observed affect states expressed through facial expression, tone of voice, body movements and other non-verbal behaviours to aspects of the physical environment. It is thought to be an advantage to use aggregated observations of the behaviour of individuals to enable the categorization of observed behaviours and environmental features into discrete and objective categories. In addition this method provides detailed information about the physical environment (Lawton 2001). There is debate about the advantages of using experts versus well-trained research assistants for observational ratings. For most of the instruments presented in the literature a thorough training period is a necessary prerequisite to rating.

A favoured design when evaluating environmental features is randomized controlled experimental studies that include two or more environmental alternatives. Participants are randomly assigned into two groups, specific outcome variables are documented in advance, and data is gathered through reliable and validated tests, observations and ratings without the awareness of the people being observed. This type of evaluation design is often not possible in research with people with dementia, mainly due to the fact that integration between residents being observed and their environments is too complex for a linear, experimentally controlled design. Therefore, it is more common to see studies using quasi-experiments and single-group studies with before and after measurements of various variables, such as those presented below.

Resident-related outcome measures

The majority of studies in the field have a quasi-experimental design, characterized by combinations of large numbers of outcome variables. Variables often used which are related to the residents' well-being include: ADLs; social and physical dependency; disorientation; rate and degree of occasions of confusion; depression; somatic health; and behavioural psychological symptoms of dementia such as wandering, aggressiveness, vocal disruption and anxiety (see for example Elmståhl, Anerstedt and Ålund 1997; Wimo *et al.* 1993).

Other studies choose to focus instead on a solitary outcome measure such as residents' actual and attempted door-openings, agitation, exit attempts, confusion, orientation ability or toileting behaviour and related issues (for example, Cohen-Mansfield, Werner and Marx 1990).

Attempts to take an objective approach are used when measuring outcomes of dementia care design such as use of drugs and physical restraints, cost of care, food consumption, amount of help needed when eating, period of sleep, residents' weights, time spent outdoors, incidents such as falls, injuries, aggression, persons missing, and mortality (for example, Namazi, Rossner and Calkins 1989).

As an attempt to learn more about the residents' perceptions of different modes of intervention in the environment some of the studies conducted have employed experimental designs. Götestam and Melin (1987) used an experimental design in their study of eating behaviour, communication and activity levels among the residents before and after implementing non-institutional dining strategies at a nursing home, as did Cooper (1999) when implementing functional colour cueing at a nursing home for dementia, measuring outcome variables including residents' experience of the legibility of the environment and the time-response of object targeting with control for visual ability. Mishima *et al.* (1994) similarly used an experimental design when measuring residents' sleeping time, behaviour disorders and melatonin secretion levels before and after exposure to morning bright light therapy, as did Passini *et al.* (2000) when studying the mobility profile of the residents at a dementia unit with the outcome measure of range of chosen destination reached.

Relative-related outcome measures

Variables commonly used to measure relatives' well-being after modification of the environment are emotional strain, attitudes towards the care in general and towards the environment, buildings and rooms specifically, and their satisfaction with unit and care (for example, Bellelli *et al.* 1998). Variables measuring the relatives' opinion or experience of the altered design include, for example, the effectiveness of the modification, or their perception of resident toileting issues (for example, Hutchinson, Leger-Krall and Wilson 1996).

Staff-related outcome measures

Outcome variables used when considering the staff perception of the effectiveness of the design programme include the influence on the residents' ADLs, on bathing problems and resident toileting issues (see for example Wimo *et al.* 1993). Outcomes related to how changes of environmental design influence staff include measures of behaviour and attitudes towards the residents, staff stress and quality of care and morale (see for example Moore 1999). Outcome measures related to workers' well-being include their general health, anxiety, depression, quality of life, guilt and grief, job satisfaction, attitudes towards care and dementia knowledge (see for example Skea and Lindsay 1996).

Concluding comments

It needs to be pointed out that when using a more qualitative design a systematic approach is equally necessary. According to Lawton (2001) this includes a specific definition of outcomes and how they fit users' needs, the use of evidence-based and best-practice knowledge from the literature together with the opinions of a reference group, and finally step-by-step guidance for observers who have the task of documenting desired and non-desired behaviours in relation to design evaluations. The evaluation notes could be sorted with reference to design-oriented and behaviour-oriented features.

'Best practice' evaluation of the effects of the environment for people with dementia

Determining how to best evaluate the effects of changes to the environment to meet users' needs is a difficult but challenging mission. Based on evidence from my own and other researchers' work, together with experiences from practical re-design projects, I have come to the following recommendations.

Designing the environment to meet users' needs requires a close but broad collaboration between representatives of all the groups involved right from the start. These collaborations should include service users together with their family members, the staff, the managing directors, architects, designers, researchers in the field and experts on specific aspects of the environment such as illumination, ventilation, landscaping and so on. See Chapters 11 and 12 for further discussion on involvement of stakeholders.

The evaluation research design should optimally include three parts: baseline, intervention and evaluation. If possible, another service should act as an experimental control in order to avoid bias effects due to concomitant factors. The specific tools and instruments to be used will depend on the resources available. If limited funds are available important information could be found using patient records, for example data on the number of falls, pharmacological treatment, duration and quality of sleep and episodes when suffering from pain. A variety of qualitative and quantitative tools and approaches may be used. For example, staff perception of workload and job satisfaction could be registered through questionnaires. Qualitative information could be collected through unstructured open interviews and through exploratory observational design.

During the analysis different perspectives can be compared and contrasted. Even though it may be difficult, it is also worthwhile to include an economic approach if possible, for example indicating that reducing falls in a nursing home could produce significant cost savings on top of decreased suffering for residents.

Caring sciences including both medical and nursing sciences are often considered as clinical sciences, with the primary aim of fighting against disease rather than promoting health. It is nevertheless evident that these two goals are closely related to each other. Evidence-based facts derived from basic research ought to be essential for the more practical clinical science. However, the way basic results are implemented in clinical practice is determined by the values and ethical considerations currently prevalent in society.

This chapter highlights some issues to consider during the environmental design process of institutions for people with dementia. These design features are of importance for the functioning and well-being of older people and people with dementia. To maximize results the starting point should be a close collaboration between architects and caring staff to ensure a better understanding of special user needs. A clear evidence-based understanding of design features is necessary to ensure effective and useful environmental improvements that will result in a decrease in environmental pressure for people with dementia. Ongoing evaluative research regarding the impact of design features is needed.

References

Antonovsky, A. (1987) *Unravelling the Mystery of Health: How People Manage Stress and Stay Well.* London: Jossey-Bass Publishers.

Baksi, A. and Cradock, S. (1998) 'What is empowerment?' *IDF Bulletin 3,* 43, 29–31.

Bellelli, G., Frisoni, G.B., Bianchetti, A., Boffelli, S., Guerrini, G.B., Scotuzzi, A., Ranieri, P., Ritondale, G., Guglielmi, L., Fusari, A., Raggi, G., Gasparotti, A., Gheza, A., Nobili, G. and Trabucchi, M. (1998) 'Special Care Units for demented patients: a multicenter study.' *The Gerontologist 38,* 456–462.

Berg, L., Buckwalter, K.C., Chafetz, P.K., Gwyther, L.P., Holmes, D., Mann Koepke, K., Lawton, M.P., Lindeman, D.A., Magaziner, J., Maslow, K., Morley, J.E., Ory, M.G., Rabins, P.V., Sloane, P.D. and Teresi, J. (1991) 'Special Care Units for patients with dementia.' *Journal of the American Gerontological Society 39,* 1229–1236.

Bowers, A.R., Meek, C. and Stewart, N. (2001) 'Illumination and reading performance in age-related macular degeneration.' *Clinical and Experimental Optometry 84,* 3, 139–147.

Brunnström, G., Sörensen, S., Alsterstad, K. and Sjöstrand, J. (2004) 'Quality of light and quality of life – the effect of lighting adaptation among people with low vision.' *Ophthalmic and Physiological Optics 24,* 4, 274–280.

Cannava, E. (1994) 'Gerodesign: safe and comfortable living spaces for older adults.' *Geriatrics 49,* 11, 45–49.

Cohen, U. and Day, K. (1993) *Contemporary Environments for People with Dementia.* Baltimore/London: The Johns Hopkins University Press.

Cohen-Mansfield, J., Werner, P. and Marx, M.S. (1990) 'The spatial distribution of agitation in agitated nursing home residents.' *Environment and Behaviour 22,* 408–419.

Cooper, B.A. (1999) 'The utility of functional colour cues: seniors' views.' *Scandinavian Journal of Caring Sciences 13,* 3, 186–192.

Day, K., Carreon, D. and Stump, C. (2000) 'The therapeutic design of environments for people with dementia: a review of the empirical research.' *Gerontologist 40,* 4, 397–416.

Dunlop, A. (1993) *Hard Architecture and Human Scale Designing for Disorientation: A Literature Review on Designing Environments for Dementia.* Stirling: Dementia Services Development Centre, University of Stirling.

Elmståhl, S., Anerstedt, L. and Ålund, O. (1997) 'How should a group-living unit for demented elderly be designed to decrease psychiatric symptoms?' *Alzheimer Disease and Associated Disorders 11,* 47–52.

Götestam, K.G. and Melin, L. (1987) 'Improving well-being for patients with senile dementia by minor changes in the ward environment.' In L. Levi (ed.) *Society, Stress and Disease.* Oxford: Oxford University Press. pp.295–297.

Gustavsson, G. (1996) *Quality of Life and Functional Capacity among Elderly with Locomotor Disability.* Licentiate thesis, Department of Caring Sciences, Linköping University, Linköping, Sweden.

Heikkinen, E., Berg, S., Schroll, M., Steen, B. and Viidik, A. (1997) 'Functional status, health and aging: the NORA study.' *Facts, Research and Intervention in Geriatrics.* Paris: Serdi.

Hillerås, P. (2000) *Well-being Among the Very Old: A Survey on a Sample Aged 90 Years or Above.* Doctoral dissertation. Department of Clinical Neuroscience and Family Medicine, Division of Geriatric Medicine, Stockholm Gerontology Research Center, Stockholm.

Hutchinson, S., Leger-Krall, S. and Wilson, H.S. (1996) 'Toileting: a bio-behavioral challenge in Alzheimer's dementia care.' *Journal of Gerontological Nursing 22,* 10, 18–27.

Karatza, M. (1995) 'The use of colours in the environment of the elderly.' *The Akon Series. Ageing in the Contemporary Society 11,* 1–102.

Kayser-Jones, J.S. (1991) 'The impact of the environment on the quality of care in nursing homes: a social-psychological perspective.' *Holistic Nursing Practice 5,* 3, 29–38.

Kelly, M. (1993) *Designing for People with Dementia in the Context of Building Standards.* Stirling: Department of Applied Social Science, University of Stirling.

Küller, R. (1991) 'Familiar design helps dementia patients cope.' In W.F.E. Preiser, J.C. Vischer and E.T. White (eds) *Design Intervention: Toward a More Humane Architecture.* New York: Van Nostrand Reinhold. pp.255–267.

Lawton, M.P. (1994) 'Quality of life in Alzheimer's disease.' *Alzheimer's Disease and Associated Disorders 8,* Supplement 3, 138–150.

Lawton, M.P. (2001) 'The physical environment of the person with Alzheimer's disease.' *Aging and Mental Health 5,* Supplement 1, SS56–64.

Lawton, M.P. and Nahemow, L. (1973) 'Ecology and the aging process.' In C. Eisdorfer and M.P. Lawton (eds) *The Psychology of Adult Development and Aging.* Washington DC: American Psychological Association. pp.619–674.

Liebowitz, B., Lawton, M.P. and Waldman, A. (1979) 'Designing for confused elderly people: lessons fron the Weiss Institute.' *American International Alzheimer's Journal 68,* 59–61.

Mishima, K., Okawa, M., Hishikawa, Y., Hozumi, S., Hori, H. and Takahashi, K. (1994) 'Morning bright light therapy for sleep and behavior disorders in elderly patients with dementia.' *Acta Psychiatry Scandinavia 89,* 1–7.

Moore, K.D. (1999) 'Dissonance in the dining room: a study of social interaction in a special care unit.' *Qualitative Health Research 9,* 133–155.

Mozley, C.G., Huxley, P. and Cordingly, L. (1999) '"Not knowing where I am doesn't mean I don't know what I like": cognitive impairment and quality of life responses in elderly people.' *International Journal of Geriatric Psychiatry 14,* 9, 776–783.

Namazi, K.H., Rossner, T. and Calkins, M. (1989) 'Visual barriers to prevent ambulatory Alzheimer's patients from exiting through an emergency door.' *The Gerontologist 29,* 699–702.

Nightingale, F. (1969) *Notes on Nursing.* New York: Dover Publications. (Original 1860.)

Orem, D.E. (1995) *Nursing: Concepts of Practice* (Fifth edition). New York: Mosby-Year Book Inc.

Passini, R., Pigot, H., Rainville, C. and Tétreault, M-H. (2000) 'Wayfinding in a nursing home for advanced dementia of the Alzheimer's type.' *Environment and Behaviour 32*, 5, 684–710.

Passini, R., Rainville, C., Marchand, N. and Joanette, Y. (1998) 'Way finding and dementia: some research findings and a new look at design.' *Journal of Architectural and Planning Research 15*, 2 (summer), 133–151.

Pastalan, L.A. (1997) *Shelter and Service Issues for Aging Populations: International Perspectives.* New York: The Haworth Press.

Ragneskog, H. (2001) *Music and Other Strategies in the Care of Agitated Individuals with Dementia.* Doctoral thesis, Gothenburg University, Gothenburg.

Sandman, P-O. (1986) *Aspects of Institutional Care of Patients with Dementia.* Doctoral dissertation, Umeå university, Umeå.

Skea, D. and Lindsay, J. (1996) 'An evaluation of two models of long-term residential care for elderly people with dementia.' *International Journal of Geriatric Psychiatry 11*, 233–241.

Watson, J. (1985) *Nursing: Human Sciences and Human Care. A Theory of Nursing.* New York: National League for Nursing.

Wijk, H. (1998) *Colour Perception in Old Age: Colour Discrimination, Colour Naming and Colour Preferences in 80-year-olds and Among Individuals Suffering from Alzheimer's Disease.* Doctoral thesis, Gothenburg University, Gothenburg.

Wijk, H. (2001) *Colour Perception in Old Age: Colour Discrimination, Colour Naming, Colour Preferences and Colour/Shape Recognition.* Doctoral thesis, Gothenburg University, Gothenburg.

Wijk, H. (in progress) 'Effects of adjustments of the physical environments for people with dementia.'

Wijk, H. and Sivik, L. (1995) 'Some aspects of colour perception among patients with Alzheimer's disease.' *Scandinavian Journal of Caring Sciences 1*, 3–9.

Wijk, H., Berg, S., Bergman, B., Börjesson Hanson, A., Sivik, L. and Steen, B. (2002) 'Color perception among the very elderly related to visual and cognitive function.' *Scandinavian Journal of Caring Sciences 16*, 91–102.

Wijk, H., Berg, S., Sivik, L. and Steen, B. (1999a) 'Colour discrimination, colour naming and colour preferences in 80-year-olds.' *Aging: Clinical Experimental Research 11*, 3, 1–10.

Wijk, H., Berg, S., Sivik, L. and Steen, B. (1999b) 'Colour discrimination, colour naming and colour preferences among patients with Alzheimer's disease.' *International Journal of Geriatric Psychiatry 14*, 1000–1005.

Wijk, H., Berg, S., Sivik, L. and Steen, B. (2001) 'Colour and form as support for picture recognition in old age.' *Aging: Clinical Experimental Research 13*, 4, 298–308.

Wimo, A., Nelvig, J., Adolfsson, R., Mattsson, B. and Sandman, P-O. (1993) 'Can changes in ward routines affect the severity of dementia? A controlled prospective study.' *International Psychogeriatrics 5*, 169–180.

Zeisel, J. (2000) 'Environmental design effects on Alzheimer symptoms in long term care residencies.' *World Hospital and Health Services 36*, 3, 2.

Chapter 7

Evaluating Long Stay Care Settings
A Study of a Life Review and Life Storybook Project

Faith Gibson, Barbara Haight and Yvonne Michel

This chapter describes the evaluation of a psychosocial intervention carried out by direct care staff (caregivers) in a variety of residential contexts and illustrates important issues relating to the evaluation of dementia care interventions. The intervention involved teaching and supporting caregivers to undertake structured life reviews and make life storybooks over an eight-week period with people diagnosed with mild to moderate dementia who resided in four statutory residential homes, a private nursing home and a not-for-profit dementia-specific housing with care facility. The evaluation was designed to measure the outcomes of the intervention for the residents and to demonstrate that caregivers, given minimal training augmented by regular supportive supervision, could implement an effective individual intervention within different types of group care settings.

Reminiscence and life review have been variously defined, and have been used in many disparate ways with undifferentiated groups of older people. Many different formats have been used to provide tangible records of people's recalled memories, including life storybooks, which have served multiple purposes ranging from identity preservation to legacy transmission. Reminiscence is a popular intervention used for enriching the lives of people of all ages but especially older people, including those who have dementia (Gibson 2004; Haight 1992; Haight and Webster

1995; Webster and Haight 2002). Reminiscence Therapy (RT) involves the discussion of past activities, events and experiences with another person or group of people, usually with the aid of tangible prompts such as photographs and other familiar items from the past, music and archive sound recordings (Woods *et al.* 2005, p.1).

Originally life storybooks were used with children who had experienced repeated disruption or trauma, often accompanied by multiple changes of location and serial parenting. They are now used in various service contexts including learning disability, palliative care and gerontology. Other formats such as memoirs, memory boxes and video films are also increasingly popular. The process of compiling a life storybook is intended to provide opportunities for forming restorative relationships and engaging in evaluative discussion with caring adults. Such books provide a lasting reference and record of significant people and places (Gibson 2004; Gillies and James 1994; Murphy and Moyes 1997; Rose and Philpot 2004; Ryan and Walker 1997). In an electronic literature search in preparation for undertaking this study no controlled evaluative studies of life storybook uses with older people who have dementia were located.

Most reminiscence undertaken with either small groups or with individuals or couples involves some elements of review and reconstruction of memories. This review element is a way of accepting, reconciling and resolving or integrating, to some extent, past pain, conflict, distress, harm endured or harm inflicted. A structured life review (the approach used in the study reported here) is a one-to-one intervention that systematically encourages a person to review the whole of life in a series of regular reminiscence discussions undertaken in private with the assistance of a facilitator. Haight's Life Review and Experiencing Form (LREF) was used to guide the life review process (Haight 1988, 1992).

There are few evaluative studies of interventions designed for people with dementia that help them to retain or regain a sense of self by means of recalling, reviewing and evaluating memories (Elford *et al.* 2005; Gibson 1994; Haight and Hendrix 1995; Hendrix and Haight 2002; Lai, Chi and Kayser-Jones 2004; Thorgrimsen, Schweitzer and Orrell 2002). Woods *et al.* (2005) have summarized the indicative if inconclusive efficacy of the few reported randomized controlled trials in their Cochrane Library review. There are even fewer studies that report outcomes from training, supporting and utilizing the skills of direct care staff in facilitating interventions like reminiscence and life review, or more importantly, how such approaches have influenced caregivers' attitudes towards residents (Bornat *et al.* 1998; Clarke, Hanson and Ross 2003). Enthusiastic practitioner accounts, however, abound concerning the benefits of reminiscence, most commonly group reminiscence, and life review with people who have dementia (Brooker and Duce 2000; Bruce and Gibson 1999a, 1999b; Woods and McKiernan 1995).

Many people who develop dementia eventually move into various kinds of residential care, which are meant to provide for graduated levels of dependency. Dementia results in a range of cognitive, social and behavioural difficulties that gradually impair verbal communication and threaten relationships. Depressed mood and loss of social skills frequently accompany cognitive losses that compromise the ability to learn or recall new or recent information, carry out normal activities of daily living, or engage in satisfying social activities (Burns, Dening and Lawlor 2002; Cherminski *et al.* 2001; Lyketsos, Steele and Baker 1997). Many people with dementia experience considerable stress, anxiety, depression and social isolation.

Caregiver stress, engendered by disruptive behaviours, frequently results in concentration on interventions designed to manage behaviour experienced as challenging and neglects interventions that promote self-esteem, preservation of personal identity, warm relationships and positive behaviours. Caregivers may fail to interpret problem behaviour as non-verbal communication and, in group living situations especially, are often discouraged from providing individualized activities or offering themselves as reassuring substitute attachment figures (Droës 1997).

A life review is an individualized response, which demands greater cognitive and organizational skills than simple reminiscence. Haight and Dias (1992) identified the crucial characteristics of a successful life review as structure, individuality, evaluation and time. Reminiscence and life review have been found to be effective for older people with depression (Bohlmeijer, Smit and Cuijpers 2004; Haight, Michel and Hendrix 1998,

2000; Watt and Cappeliez 2000; Woods 2004). Butler (2002) noted similarities between life review and psychotherapy both being processes designed to review the past so as to make the present more comprehensible and the future less fearful. In reminiscence and life review, authority and control remain with the person (Dunn, Haight and Hendrix 2002). Mills and Coleman (2002) and Coleman, Hautamaki and Podolskij (2002) noted the efficacy of reminiscence and life review as communication tools and as means of achieving reconciliation, resolution and generativity or accepting and making sense of memories of past painful experiences. Kasl-Godley and Gatz (2000) believe that the available evidence shows that life review and reminiscence provide people with mild to moderate dementia with better inter-personal connections and more satisfying relationships than any other intervention.

Description of the project

A small controlled pilot study involved 30 older people with dementia, two researchers and 14 residential caregivers and was undertaken in Northern Ireland over eight weeks. The intervention combined individual structured life reviews based on verbal reminiscence and recall with the compilation of simple life storybooks. The project aimed to evaluate the effectiveness of this intervention with a small number of older people diagnosed with mild to moderate dementia who were no longer capable of living in their own homes. It sought to assist people to value themselves by valuing their recalled past lives and by so doing improve their quality of life. The primary objective was to evaluate the outcomes of the intervention in terms of:

- decreased depression and improved mood
- improved behaviour
- increased functioning in activities of daily living
- improved communication.

Secondary objectives were: to enrich the caring environments by offering a new experience to residents, equipping the caregivers with new inter-personal communication skills and producing a tangible record of people's lives to be used as a tool for ongoing conversation, memory jogging and information provision.

Familiar caregivers undertook life review sessions and compiled the life storybooks. These weekly reminiscing conversations were loosely structured by using the LREF (Haight 1991) which encouraged a systematic review of the whole of life through childhood, adolescence, adult life and late life. Each person was encouraged to reflect upon each life stage and on their life overall. The life storybook compiled in a loose-leaf binder was a simple chronological compilation of personally relevant photographs and memorabilia together with short descriptive captions quoting the person's own words.

Consent

The criteria for inclusion in the study were a diagnosis of dementia, sufficient residual speech to be able to engage in the weekly sessions and a willingness to participate (see Box 7.1 for characteristics of the participants). Participants required sufficient mental capacity to give informed consent according to the ethical protocol of the Medical University of South Carolina based upon the Belmont Report (1979). One author administered the Mini Mental Status Examination (MMSE) to all subjects to determine competence to consent. Another author then met each participant, again explained the purpose and process of the study and obtained written consent. Whenever possible these initial testing and consent interviews were undertaken in the presence of a familiar caregiver. All participants freely signed their own consent forms except one woman whose mental capacity score fell below the required level (12 points on the MMSE). Her younger brother gave proxy consent.

Methodology and evaluation

A pre and post-test study design was used (Pierce 2005). Residents in the experimental group undertook the reminiscence/life review sessions while the control group continued to receive their usual care. Demographic and medical data was gathered from the participant's records and augmented by the caregivers. Box 7.2 shows the list of standardized measures used.

Box 7.1 Characteristics of the participants

- 20% were men, 80% were women.

- Participant ages ranged from 65 to 99 and averaged 82 years.

- All were mobile and 84% considered they were in good health despite numerous age-related physical infirmities.

- Almost a third reported having been alcohol dependent and several had enduring functional mental health problems.

- 74% were widowed, 7% still married, 6% divorced and 13% had never married.

- 48% of participants had attended elementary school only, 28% attended secondary school and 24% had undertaken some further education or trade-related training.

- The majority (77%) had regular contact with their families but only one third considered they had a safe and trusted confidant.

Box 7.2 Standardized measures used in this study

Cognition: Mini Mental State Examination (MMSE) (Folstein, Folstein and McHugh 1975). The MMSE was used both as a baseline measure and at the post-test stage as an indicator of level of cognitive functioning.

Communication: Communication Observation Scale (COS) (Tappen 2000) – designed to measure verbal and non-verbal communication.

Depression: Cornell Scale for Depression in Dementia (CSDD) (Alexopoulos, Abrams and Young 1998) – a test of direct observation designed to assess depressive symptoms in dementia. Completed by caregivers.

Mood: Alzheimer's Mood Scale (Tappen 2000) – a 53-item adjective test list designed for caregivers to rate the mood of care receivers during the preceding week.

Independence: Functional Independence Measure (FIM) (Granger *et al.* 1990) – designed to measure functioning regardless of the underlying pathology or clinical background of the test administrator.

Behaviour: Alzheimer's Memory and Behaviour Checklist (Teri *et al.* 1992) – a 24-item list of observable behaviour problems completed by the caregivers.

Training and support of the caregivers delivering the intervention

An integral part of this project was a desire to equip direct caregivers with new inter-personal skills in the hope that the intervention might continue to be used in these facilities after the project was completed. Consequently the researchers did not carry out the intervention, a common procedure in research projects, but rather trained and supported caregivers to do so. The managers of the six facilities nominated caregivers and possible residents. The latter were randomly assigned to either an experimental or control group. Initial training was followed by weekly supervision sessions for the caregivers with the researchers in each facility. All agreed to tape-record the reminiscence sessions, to make the tapes available for supervision, and to seek material from the family carers to assist in compiling the life storybooks.

Box 7.3 sets out the characteristics of the caregivers.

Box 7.3 Characteristics of the caregivers

- One male and 13 female caregivers.
- Nine caregivers perceived themselves as having volunteered to participate in the project while five designated themselves as 'conscripts'.
- Caregivers were aged 24 to 57 years with an average age of 38.
- Years in care work ranged from 2 to 25 and averaged 12 years. Years of employment in their present facility ranged from 2 to 17 and averaged six years.
- Eight had undertaken formal care-related training since leaving school.
- One held a social work qualification, one held certificates in social care and counselling, four either had or were currently studying for National Vocational Qualifications in Care at Levels II or III, one was a State Enrolled Nurse and one had a certificate in therapeutic arts.
- Two were managers, four were senior care assistants, one divided her time between being an activity officer and a care assistant and seven were graded as care assistants.
- None of the caregivers had previous experience of undertaking individual structured life reviews/life storybooks, although six had done basic reminiscence training. One senior carer had substantial experience of leading small reminiscence groups.

Process or internal evaluation

Regrettably no systematic attempt was made to ascertain the attitudes of the caregivers towards the project at the pre-test stage. Halfway through the project each researcher independently rated the caregivers looking at their understanding of the project, openness, listening, empathizing and responding skills, relationship building, pleasurable engagement and responsiveness to supervision. At the end of the project, caregivers completed a short anonymous questionnaire about the project and their participation in it.

The questionnaire completed at the end of the project asked the caregivers retrospectively about their initial response when first asked to become involved in the project and their response after having been involved. Initial responses were almost equally divided between reports of positive and negative feelings. Feelings at the post-project stage were overwhelmingly positive for the majority of 11 although three expressed trenchant reservations. Two caregivers from the same facility described themselves at the end as 'less enthusiastic' and 'more wary' while a third reported the project as only 'moderately interesting – a sort of formalized reminiscence which was not difficult but time consuming'. The voluntary participation of caregivers and their willingness and capacity to scrutinize their inter-personal involvement with residents emerged as important issues.

A recurring theme was the issue of having insufficient time to undertake the weekly sessions despite the initial assurances of the facility managers that time would be made available. Although expressing very positive responses overall, the majority mentioned that lack of dedicated time would deter them from undertaking future life reviews/life storybooks. All believed that the intervention could be helpful in their work setting in the future and most would like to use it again if the time issue could be resolved. Eight commented that staffing levels would need to be adjusted and such individualized work would need to be explicitly recognized as a part of a caregiver's regular workload so that colleagues accorded it respect.

The need to explain the life review/life storybook process more fully to all members of staff of residential facilities was identified as essential and some suggested that it would be desirable for several members of staff to be trained in the intervention. Three caregivers suggested the intervention should either be incorporated into initial assessments prior to admission or should be linked to the first review (6–12 weeks after admission) in order to inform care planning and assist an individual's induction into residential care. Most mentioned introductory training and regular group discussions as essential means for providing ongoing support for staff undertaking such an intervention.

Being asked to tape-record interviews and participate in weekly supervision sessions based largely upon these recordings was a novel experience for all caregivers who were asked what they thought about the teaching and learning process and how they might wish to change it. Ten commented that the initial training session was well set out, the supervision was well organized and valuable and that the intervention was 'easy to learn'. Two caregivers thought that the initial training session was too short and provided insufficient preparation, beliefs which contrasted starkly with another's comment – 'I wouldn't change anything.'

Eleven caregivers said they valued the supervision while three were ambivalent. Responsibility for listening to each worker's tape alternated between the two researchers who then participated jointly in most supervision discussions. Although all staff were used to being supervised, none was accustomed to such frequent supervision or to the closeness of scrutiny of their interactions with residents that the audio tape recordings made possible. The researcher who had listened to the tape took the lead in providing initial feedback with both contributing freely to the ensuing discussion in order to model a collaborative working relationship (Kadushin and Harkness 2002). In the housing with care facility, group supervision predominated but was augmented by tandem or individual supervision according to caregiver availability. In other locations, individual and paired supervisions were held according to the personal preferences and availability of caregivers (Gibson 2004).

The three caregivers described as ambivalent found the close weekly scrutiny of their interviews and subsequent discussion problematic. The reasons for this varied for each person but raised important questions about how best to support staff when implementing a new intervention such as this. The most experienced reminiscence worker of all found shifting from group to individual work difficult and remained unenthusiastic about working intensively in a more structured way with an individual resident. She experienced supervision as inappropriately critical. Her colleague in the same facility felt that her resident made insufficient progress to justify the time invested. Both residents allocated to these caregivers had long-standing, intractable mental health and substance dependency problems. One became more demanding of personal attention as the project progressed and the caregiver and other staff colleagues were quick to attribute this person's demanding behaviour to the project.

The third worker, a conscript, also experienced supervision as uncomfortably intrusive and unduly critical. This caregiver remained equivocal about the value of talking about the past and sceptical of the resident's capacity to respond. Completion of the life review/life storybook was delayed because of holiday arrangements. The early supervision sessions for these three caregivers proceeded on the basis of verbal reports because the tapes were not forthcoming – possibly indicating early anxiety or ambivalence about participation. Another factor that compounded their negative responses was the failure of the three relevant families to provide photographs. The request for material, however, succeeded in re-establishing contact between one woman and her daughter after a considerable lapse of time – an impressive achievement that the caregiver was reluctant to attribute to the work that she had done.

It would seem, therefore, that a number of structural and personal reasons contributed towards the low level of satisfaction experienced by a minority of caregivers. The researchers who felt constrained by the time-bounded nature of this project no doubt also contributed. The project was undoubtedly demanding of caregivers, most of whom, although experienced residential care workers, lacked prior training in the counselling skills required to emphasize and to listen to the painful life experiences inevitably raised by residents.

Caregivers needed considerable support and encouragement to explore the detail of residents' stories. Initially they perceived themselves as 'nosey' and 'intrusive' when asking questions and, although some were natural listeners, most found it difficult to stay with overt expressions of pain and sadness. Initially most were eager to move the conversation into less demanding territory. Over time the audio tapes provided evidence of improved pacing within sessions, of growing skill in prompting more detailed recall and adjusting to the residents' variable energy levels, and of considerable excitement and pleasure when coherent recollections and entertaining stories emerged.

Caregivers displayed increasing ability to use the questions from the LREF as gentle probes, as invitations to talk and to share memories rather than as ammunition for conducting a quick-fire inquisition. Most reported some reluctance to explore the topic of sexuality and were surprised at the ease with which the older people talked about this aspect of their lives. The physical and intellectual disabilities with which the participants were contending posed considerable challenges to the caregivers who began to learn new ways of listening, talking and responding. They were able to build on their existing relationships and use material gathered in the sessions as the basis for engaging in opportunistic reminiscence-related conversations in between sessions.

Overall, caregivers were enthusiastic, although not uncritical. They were generous in the time and energy they devoted to the project and united, with one exception, in their strong conviction that they had come to know the residents in a new and deeper way. They were able to recognize and appreciate their own developing inter-personal skills of empathetic attentive listening, reflecting and attending (Shulman 1999). All but one unreservedly believed that the residents had profited from the experience of recounting and reviewing their life stories, that the residents valued the life storybooks that had been created, and that they and the residents had achieved improved communication and enriched relationships (Hargie, Saunders and Dickson 2002). The realization that so many members of care staff with brief initial preparation, and with continuing support, were able to achieve so much is a tribute to their motivation, skill and commitment. It indicates considerable potential, providing adequate time could be made available, for caregivers to use such an intervention, which is able to transform the nature of resident–caregiver relationships within varied care settings.

Evaluation of the responses of families

For resource and logistical reasons this project excluded relatives from directly participating in the life review/life storybook process, although couples' reminiscence and life review has been used to good effect (Kurokawa 1998). Nor did it intentionally attempt to collect relatives' views about the project's influence. Some staff members, however, incidentally reported that family members welcomed the additional personal attention the project afforded their relatives. Most were eager to provide photographs and other information, and the three who did not seemed to be more indifferent than hostile. Family members appeared to value the life books, as indicated by the sister of one man who died shortly after completing his book. At his funeral she sought out the caregiver who had worked with her brother saying how pleased she was that although her brother had died 'we still have Jim's book'. When a 95-year-old woman proudly displayed her book to her son he graphically described his mother's pleasure and excitement by volunteering 'Mum's eyes are dancing in her head'.

Outcome or external evaluation

Statistical analysis of the scores from the different measures used within the evaluation showed a significant improvement in the well-being of the participants with dementia (see Table 7.1). Statistically significant gains over time were found for the experimental group on measures of cognition, depression, mood and communication which indicated that the people who had engaged in the life review/life storybook intervention benefited greatly from this experience. The improved MMSE scores possibly indicate that the residents in the experimental group profited from the increased social and intellectual stimulation arising from individual weekly reminiscence sessions. The chronologically structured focus of the recall stimulated participants to organize and rehearse their memories both as a consequence of sessions and in anticipation of future sessions. This continuing stimulation is illustrated for example by one man who asked his daughter to bring in a suitcase full of family photographs, most

Table 7.1 Means, standard deviations and gain scores for outcome measures

Group	Number	Pre-test mean (SD)	Post-test mean (SD)	Gain score
Mini Mental Status Exam (MMSE)				
E1	14	16.93 (5.85)	20.29 (4.70)	+ 3.36
C1	16	18.56 (5.47)	14.65 (5.58)	– 3.91
Cornell Scale for Depression in Dementia (CSDD)				
E1	15	10.40 (4.69)	6.08 (4.27)	– 4.32
C1	16	11.06 (7.00)	11.71 (8.72)	+ 0.65
Alzheimer's Mood Scale N(AMS neg)				
E1	15	54.93 (12.68)	39.14 (6.85)	– 15.79
C1	15	58.38 (21.02)	54.07 (23.80)	– 4.31
Alzheimer's Mood Scale P(AMS pos)				
E1	15	86.40 (16.29)	101.43 (15.40)	+ 15.03
C1	15	81.73 (20.48)	81.94 (21.10)	+ 0.21
Functional Independence Measure (FIM)				
E1	15	94.69 (23.81)	107.64 (20.81)	+ 12.95
C1	15	88.69 (20.26)	90.47 (31.39)	+ 1.78
Communication Observation Scale for Cognitively Impaired (COS)				
E1	15	26.60 (5.36)	30.93 (2.02)	+ 4.33
C1	15	28.50 (4.10)	23.24 (4.12)	– 5.26
Memory and Behaviour Problems Checklist (MBS)				
E1	15	30.73 (9.57)	22.42 (11.91)	– 8.31
C1	15	31.94 (13.72)	36.24 (28.62)	+ 4.30

E1: experimental group
C1: control group
SD: standard deviation

of which she had never seen before, and staff observed them sharing many happy recollections together during several visits.

The improvement in post-test Communication Observation Scale scores indicated a considerable gain for the experimental group and marked deterioration in control group scores, possibly reflecting the value of regular practice for conserving and improving competence in conversation.

The Cornell Scale for Depression in Dementia scores showed significant decreases for the experimental group while remaining level for the control group. This improvement in depression accords with previous findings for nursing home populations without dementia who undertook life reviews (Haight *et al.* 1998, 2000). The decrease in scores suggests that recalling and rehearsing old memories, some of which may be painful, decreases depression, even for people who are coping with dementia (Mills and Coleman 2002). The Alzheimer's Mood Scale scores also showed a significant increase in the good mood scores for the life review group with the control group showing little change. Both groups showed almost equal but not statistically significant improvement on the Functional Independence Measure and on the Memory and Behaviour Problems Checklist.

No attempt was made to quantitatively assess the impact of the preparation of the life storybooks on either residents or caregivers or to disentangle the relative contributions of the life reviews and life storybooks. Subjective reports indicated that the books were much valued and it is hoped that they will continue to be used as a focus for future conversation and as 'passports' should their owners be hospitalized or need to transfer to another facility. Most caregivers enjoyed compiling the books although more time was needed than originally anticipated.

The absence of personal memorabilia presented considerable obstacles, not always successfully overcome, although new and alternative photographs compensated in small ways for this lack. This aspect of the project identified the importance of encouraging families to preserve cherished objects and significant memorabilia, including photographs of people and places (Chaudhury 2003; Sherman 1991), and to ensure that cherished memorabilia is available and accessible to people, not withstanding those with dementia, who are admitted to care.

Summative evaluation

This small controlled pilot study demonstrated that it is possible to use standardized psychometric measures to evaluate the impact of an intervention such as structured life review/life storybook work with older people who have dementia in long-term residential facilities. It also showed that caregivers, given adequate induction training, support and time, are able to implement such an intervention. While residents benefited, the caregivers also enjoyed the closer relationships, detailed knowledge, improved understanding and enriched communication that developed as consequences of this intervention. The intervention was undertaken using an opportunistic sample, but the allocation of subjects to either an experimental or a control group was randomized within each facility, and the similarities between both groups at the pre-test stage were established. Therefore it is not unreasonable, given the significant statistical outcomes achieved on four of the six measures used, to conclude that the intervention contributed to the outcomes achieved. For the experimental group, statistically significant differences at post-test were obtained on measures of cognition, depression, mood and communication. It is acknowledged, however, that during the intervention the presence and novelty of the project may have influenced the general ethos of the residential facilities in unidentified ways and the regular supervision of the caregivers involved may have introduced additional uncontrolled variables. It is not possible to say definitively which aspects of the intervention contributed to the improved scores. It should be noted that the statistical significance of the figures is based on small sample sizes and a bigger sample would strengthen the conclusions drawn here.

Perhaps undivided, regular personal attention was as important as the cognitive stimulation provided by the LREF-based reminiscence and recall processes linked to the construction of the life storybooks. The capacity of the participants, although having dementia, to review their lives to some extent more or less systematically, both stage-by-stage and overall, and to articulate their stories, was impressive. They enjoyed the undivided individual attention and demonstrated in many small ways that they appreciated and valued their life storybooks. Disentangling the relative importance of each aspect of the project as well as comparing this intervention with other individual and group psychosocial interventions must await future research.

The evaluation involved pre and post-test methodology and the study of both process and outcome aspects of a time-limited intervention. Two independent researchers delivered the initial brief training of the residential caregivers involved and their weekly supervisions. They also carried out the pre and post-testing and assisted in various ways with the creation of the life storybooks. This multiplicity of roles carried by the researchers as well as by the familiar caregivers, not entirely desirable in the interests of scientific detachment, represents one of the many factors likely to constrain the evaluation of psychosocial interventions utilized with people who have dementia in residential care settings. The evaluation demonstrated positive outcomes for participants and caregivers. It identified the major constraints of time and workload management which resource providers and managers must face if wishing to implement a life review/life storybook intervention in residential care provision.

The psychometric tools or instruments used in the evaluation of this project provided evidence of the effectiveness of the life review/life storybook intervention with the residents. The less rigorous questionnaires, interview tapes and subjective assessments of the researchers provided multiple sources of qualitative information about the attitudes, competence and levels of satisfaction with the project of the staff who implemented the intervention.

The study adds further data to a slowly accumulating body of evidence of the effectiveness of psychosocial or non-pharmacological interventions for people with dementia. It is noteworthy for having utilized a life review/life storybook approach with residents in three different types of group care contexts, delivered by members of direct care staff. Residents enjoyed the process, which for them resulted in significant improvements in cognition, depression, mood and communication as well as the production of a tangible product of a simple life storybook. Most of the care staff involved also derived benefit from the experience. It is possible to speculate that the increased job satisfaction for staff and enhanced resident– carer communication arising from the intervention had the potential to influence the care environments beyond the life of this project.

The evaluation approach used, however, focused only on capturing short-term change within individuals. It was not constructed to address changes in the context of care, although it quickly became apparent that structures, policies, resources, rigidities in roles and responsibilities as well as attitudes of work colleagues would either facilitate or obstruct future applications of this or similar approaches. To achieve and then to sustain effective change for individual residents, broader structural and personnel concerns related to the contexts within which older people with dementia live must also become a focus for attention, and consequently a crucial part of the evaluation process.

References

Alexopoulos, G.S., Abrams, R.C. and Young, R.C. (1998) 'Cornell scale for depression in dementia.' *Biological Psychiatry 23*, 271–284.

Belmont Report (1979) *Ethical Principles and Guidelines for the Protection of Human Subjects for Research.* Washington, DC: Department of Health, Education and Welfare.

Bohlmeijer, E., Smit, E. and Cuijpers, P. (2004) 'Effects of reminiscence and life review on late-life depression: a meta analysis.' *International Journal of Geriatric Psychiatry 18*, 12, 1088–1094.

Bornat, J., Chamberlayne, P., Chant, L. and Pavey, S. (eds) (1998) *Redefining Reminiscence in Care Settings.* London: University of East London, Centre for Biography in Social Policy.

Brooker, D.J.R. and Duce, L. (2000) 'Well-being and activity in dementia: a comparison of group reminiscence therapy, structured goal-directed activity and unstructured time.' *Aging and Mental Health 4*, 356–360.

Bruce, E. and Gibson, F. (1999a) 'Stimulating communication: project evaluation Part 1.' *Journal of Dementia Care 7*, 2, 18–19.

Bruce, E. and Gibson, F. (1999b) 'Remembering yesterday: having fun, making friends: project evaluation Part 2.' *Journal of Dementia Care 7*, 3, 28–29.

Burns, A., Dening, T. and Lawlor, B. (2002) *Clinical Guidelines in Old Age Psychiatry.* London: Martin Dunitz.

Butler, R. (2002) 'The life review.' *Journal of Geriatric Psychiatry 35*, 1, 7–10.

Chaudhury, H. (2003) 'Quality of life and place therapy.' In R.J. Scheidt and P.G. Windley (eds) *Physical Environments and Aging: Critical Contributions of M. Powell Lawton to Theory and Practice.* Binghampton, New York: Haworth Press. pp.85–103.

Cherminski, E., Petracca, G., Sabe, L., Kremer, J. and Starkstein, S. (2001) 'The specificity of depressive symptoms in patients with Alzheimer's disease.' *American Journal of Psychiatry 158*, 1, 68–72.

Clarke, A., Hanson, E.J. and Ross, E.H. (2003) 'Seeing the person behind the patient: enhancing the care of older people using a biographical approach.' *Journal of Clinical Nursing 12*, 697–706.

Coleman, P.G., Hautamaki, A. and Podolskij, A. (2002) 'Trauma, reconciliation and generativity. Stories told by European war veterans.' In J.D. Webster and B.K. Haight (eds) *Critical Advances in Reminiscence Work: From Theory to Application.* New York: Springer-Verlag. pp.218–232.

Droës, R.M. (1997) 'Psychological treatment for demented patients: an overview of methods and effects.' In B.M.L. Miesen and G.M.M. Jones (eds) *Care-giving in Dementia: Research and Applications 2.* London: Routledge.

Dunn, P., Haight, B.K. and Hendrix, S. (2002) 'Power dynamics in the interpersonal life review dyad.' *Journal of Geriatric Psychiatry 35*, 1, 77–94.

Elford, H., Wilson, F., McKee, K.J., Chung, M.C., Bolton, G. and Goudie, F. (2005) 'Psychosocial benefits of solitary reminiscence writing: an exploratory study.' *Aging and Mental Health 9*, 4, 305–314.

Folstein, M.F., Folstein, S.E. and McHugh, P. (1975) 'Mini Mental State: a practical method for grading the cognitive state of patients for the clinician.' *Journal of Psychiatric Research 12*, 189–198.

Gibson, F. (1994) 'What can reminiscence contribute to people with dementia?' In J. Bornat (ed.) *Reminiscence Reviewed: Perspectives, Evaluations and Achievements.* Buckingham: Open University Press. pp.46–60.

Gibson, F. (2004) *The Past in the Present: Using Reminiscence in Health and Social Care.* Baltimore: Health Professions Press.

Gillies, C. and James, A. (1994) *Reminiscence Work with Old People.* London: Chapman Hall.

Granger, C.V., Cotter, A.C., Hamilton, B., Fiedler, R.C. and Hens, M. (1990) 'Functional assessment scales: a study of persons with multiple sclerosis.' *Archives of Rehabilitation, Physical Medical 71*, 870–875.

Haight, B.K. (1988) 'The therapeutic role of a structured life review process in homebound elderly subjects.' *Journal of Gerontology: Psychological Sciences 43*, 2, 40–44.

Haight, B.K. (1991) 'Reminiscing: the state of the art as a basis for practice.' *International Journal of Aging and Human Development 33*, 1, 1–32.

Haight, B.K. (1992) 'Long-term effects of a structured life review process.' *Journal of Gerontology 47*, 312–315.

Haight, B.K. and Dias, J.K. (1992) 'Examining key variables in selected reminiscing modalities.' *International Psychogeriatrics 4*, Supplement 2, 279–290.

Haight, B.K. and Hendrix, S. (1995) 'An integrated review of reminiscence.' In B.K. Haight and J.D. Webster (eds) *The Art and Science of Reminiscing: Theory, Research, Methods, and Applications.* Washington, DC: Taylor and Francis. pp.3–9.

Haight, B.K. and Webster, J.D. (1995) *The Art and Science of Reminiscing: Theory, Research, Methods, and Applications.* Washington, DC: Taylor and Francis.

Haight, B.K., Michel, Y. and Hendrix, S. (1998) 'Life review: preventing despair in newly relocated nursing home residents short and long term effects.' *International Journal of Aging and Human Development 47*, 2, 119–142.

Haight, B.K., Michel, Y. and Hendrix, S. (2000) 'The extended effects of the life review in nursing home residents.' *International Journal of Aging and Human Development 50*, 2, 151–168.

Hargie, O., Saunders, C. and Dickson, D. (2002) *Social Skills in Interpersonal Communication*. London: Routledge.

Hendrix, S. and Haight, B.K. (2002) 'A continued review of reminiscence.' In J.D. Webster and B.K. Haight (eds) *Critical Advances in Reminiscence Work: From Theory to Application*. New York: Springer. pp.3–29.

Kadushin, A. and Harkness, D. (2002) *Supervision in Social Work*. New York: Columbia University Press.

Kasl-Godley, J. and Gatz, M. (2000) 'Psychosocial interventions for individuals with dementia: an integration of theory, therapy and a clinical understanding of dementia.' *Clinical Psychology Review 20*, 6, 755–782.

Kurokawa, Y. (1998) 'Couple reminiscence with Japanese dementia patients.' In P. Schweitzer (ed.) *Reminiscence in Dementia Care*. London: Age Exchange. pp.108–112.

Lai, C.K.Y., Chi, I. and Kayser-Jones, J.A. (2004) 'A randomised control trial of a specific reminiscence approach to promote the well-being of nursing home residents with dementia.' *Journal of International Psychogeriatrics 16*, 33–49.

Lyketsos, C.G., Steele, C. and Baker, L. (1997) 'Major and minor depression in Alzheimer's disease: prevalence and impact.' *The Journal of Neuropsychiatry and Clinical Neurosciences 9*, 556–561.

Mills, M. and Coleman, P.G. (2002) 'Using reminiscence and life review with older people: a psychodynamic approach.' *Journal of Geriatric Psychiatry: A Multidisciplinary Journal of Mental Health and Aging 35*, 1, 63–76.

Murphy, C. and Moyes, M. (1997) 'Life story work.' In M. Marshall (ed.) *State of the Art in Dementia Care*. London: Centre for Policy on Ageing. pp.149–153.

Pierce, T. (2005) 'Evaluation issues in group work.' In B.K. Haight and F. Gibson (eds) *Burnside's Working with Older Adults: Group Process and Techniques* (Fourth edition). Boston: Jones and Bartlett. pp.469–480.

Rose, R. and Philpot, T. (2004) *The Child's Own Story: Life Story Work with Traumatized Children*. London: Jessica Kingsley Publishers.

Ryan, T. and Walker, R. (1997) *Life Story Work*. London: British Agencies for Adoption and Fostering.

Sherman, E. (1991) 'Reminiscentia: cherished objects as memorabilia in late life reminiscence.' *International Journal of Aging and Human Development 38*, 89–100.

Shulman, L. (1999) *The Skills of Helping Individuals, Groups and Communities*. Istaca, IL: Peacock Press.

Tappen, R. (2000) (Personal communication).

Teri, L., Truax, P., Logsdon, R., Uomoto, J., Zarit, S. and Vitaliano, P. (1992) 'Assessment of behavioral problems in dementia: the revised memory and behavior problems checklist.' *Psychology and Aging 7*, 622–631.

Thorgrimsen, L., Schweitzer, P. and Orrell, M. (2002) 'Evaluating reminiscence for people with dementia: a pilot study.' *Arts in Psychotherapy 65*, 6, 283–287.

Watt, L.M. and Cappeliez, P. (2000) 'Integrative and instrumental reminiscence therapies for depression in older adults: intervention strategies and treatment effectiveness.' *Aging and Mental Health 4*, 2, 166–177.

Webster, J. and Haight, B.K. (2002) *Critical Advances in Reminiscence Work: From Theory to Application.* New York: Springer.

Woods, B. (2004) 'Review: reminiscence and life review are effective therapies for depression in the elderly.' *Evidence-Based Mental Health 7*, 81.

Woods, B. and McKiernan, F. (1995) 'Evaluating the impact of reminiscence on older people with dementia.' In B.K. Haight and J.D. Webster (1995) *The Art and Science of Reminiscing: Theory, Research, Methods, and Applications.* Washington, DC: Taylor and Francis. pp.233–242.

Woods, B., Spector, A., Jones, C., Orrell, M. and Davis, S. (2005) 'Reminiscence therapy for dementia.' In *The Cochrane Database of Systematic Reviews, Issue 3.* Oxford: Wiley Inter Science.

Chapter 8

Evaluating Long Stay Settings
Reflections on the Process with Particular Reference to Dementia Care Mapping

Anthea Innes and Fiona Kelly

This chapter draws on our experiences of evaluating long stay dementia care settings: both care homes and hospital wards. We begin by providing a short overview of the Dementia Care Mapping method and our rationale for using it as a tool to evaluate long stay dementia care settings. We then discuss the process of evaluating dementia care and our reflections on the strengths and limitations of the method for this purpose. We conclude by suggesting that, when evaluating long stay care, there are a number of other techniques that could be used to enhance the usefulness of Dementia Care Mapping. As such, we advocate the use of a 'tool kit' when approaching the task of evaluating long stay dementia care.

Why use Dementia Care Mapping?

There is a growing number of publications relating to the Dementia Care Mapping (DCM) method. They range from discussions about its suitability as a tool for research (see Brooker, in press, for review) and practice (e.g. Adams 1996; Innes 2002a) to accounts of research studies where DCM has been one of the tools used (e.g. Innes and Surr 2001; Kuhn, Fulton and Endelmann 2004). The literature includes personal accounts from practitioners about their experiences of using DCM (e.g. Beavis 1998; Kuhn and

Verity 2002; Muller-Hergl 2004) and two edited collections dedicated to DCM (Brooker, Edwards and Benson 2004; Innes 2003a). This growth in the number of DCM-related publications reflects a growing increase in usage of the method not only in the UK but also internationally (Edwards 2005). So what may attract evaluators of long stay dementia care settings to use DCM? The attraction may lie in its apparent ability to evaluate the care setting in its entirety. A typical map will be conducted over a six-hour time period. Only public and communal areas are observed and not bedrooms or bathrooms. During this time, four coding frames are used to record the lives of up to ten people with dementia in five-minute intervals or time frames (Bradford Dementia Group 1997). The four coding frames are:

- *Well and ill-being values (WIB).* There are six codes to choose from. These range from −5 to +5 and are assigned to each five-minute time frame.

- *Behaviour category codes (BCC).* There are BCCs roughly equating to each letter of the alphabet. Ranging from sleep (N: land of nod) to verbal communications (A: articulation), eating and drinking (F: food and drink) and expressive activities (E: expression).

- *Personal detractions (PD).* There are 17 types of PD, for example treachery, objectification, infantilization, mockery. Each form of PD is assigned a level of severity ranging from mild, to moderate, severe and very severe.

- *Positive events (PE).* This coding frame is the least developed in the seventh edition of the DCM manual used in our studies. It is based on Kitwood's concept of positive person work (1997) and includes times when staff demonstrate skill and sensitivity that enhances well-being or prevents or contains ill-being, for example acknowledging an individual's distress or encouraging and enabling an individual to maintain abilities and skills.

Our reasons for using DCM relate to its unique framework providing information about:

- the level of well or ill-being of individuals with dementia in a care setting

- what people with dementia do during an observation period (six hours)

- instances where the person with dementia is 'put down' in some way

- instances where staff demonstrate aspects of what is known as positive person work (Kitwood 1997).

The use of this framework allows for structured observations of key aspects of the quality of care received by people with dementia. The snapshot (six hours) provides an overview of the care received during the observation period and thus becomes a baseline for comparison with future observation periods. It also allows for a comparison of observations on different days of the week where different activities may be available and different staff may be on duty.

The studies

As part of our individual PhD research projects we elected to use DCM as one tool to provide information about the care provided to people with dementia in care homes (Innes) and long stay hospital wards (Kelly).

The aim of the care home study was to systematically explore the process of culture change in three care homes in England (Innes 2000). This involved the design and delivery of a student-centred learning training programme to help equip staff with knowledge about dementia care and incorporated assignments designed to help them to implement aspects of person-centred care into their daily practice through the development of life history work and care planning. This is discussed in detail elsewhere (Innes 2002b). Dementia Care Mapping feedback sessions provided an opportunity for ongoing dialogue with staff about their care practices before, during and following the completion of the training programme.

The aim of the hospital ward study is to explore whether creative sessions facilitate expression of selfhood (Sabat 2002) thereby improving the well-being of people with dementia in long-term care. This study began in May 2004, is due to be completed in May 2007, and is set within three wards of a large city psychiatric hospital. Initially DCM was used to add focus to ethnographic fieldwork and to produce a comparative time sequence within which to evaluate the impact of creative sessions on those who participated in them. A series of six-hour maps was carried out on participants whose next of kin had given consent and who themselves had agreed with the researcher's request to observe their day. These maps spanned four weeks for each participant and were carried out on the one day in each week that the art and occupational therapists came to the ward to provide creative sessions for the participants. The data obtained from the creative sessions were embedded in each six-hour map and allowed the researcher to compare participants' well-being and self-expression during the creative sessions with the hours before each session and the hours following it.

Along with keeping ethnographic field notes and carrying out DCM, the researcher also sought ethical approval and permission from next of kin to video-record participants as they took part in the creative sessions. The process of gaining consent from participants with dementia followed Dewing (2002). Dewing proposed that many people with dementia are pleased to be asked to take part in research, feeling that they are being viewed as capable people again. She argued that if DCM is to adhere to its person-centred principles then the process of gaining consent should be inclusionary. As such, information needs to be given in 'non-cognitively threatening ways': in manageable chunks with the use of props when appropriate (Dewing 2002, p.159). Consents were sought from those who participated in the creative sessions on each occasion by showing them the video recorder and how it worked and asking whether they would mind if the researcher took a 'moving picture' of them. All those approached were eager to participate. One of the rationales for using a video recording method was to capture the subtleties of interaction (e.g. vocal and visual communication) and action (e.g. mime, work-like or intellectual activity) that might be missed using observation alone. The video footage was analysed using DCM, although this proved problematic as will be discussed further below.

Reflections on the process of evaluating dementia care

The process of evaluating long stay care through DCM ideally involves providing briefing information for care staff, maintaining an open process when the evaluator is observing the care setting, delivering prompt feedback to staff after the evaluation, providing information about what was observed and creating the opportunity for discussion of observations and care practices. These key stages of the DCM evaluation process reflect the process of evaluations using other techniques (Rossi, Lipsey and Freeman 2004). We reflect on each of these stages in turn.

Briefing staff

Briefing sessions were scheduled with the help of the care settings' management teams, to allow the evaluators to explain about the method and the purpose of the evaluations, and for the evaluators to meet the staff teams and to hear their concerns and viewpoints about the planned observations. Ethnographic field notes on the briefing sessions, where the evaluator reflects on the briefing sessions, can provide useful further data with which to evaluate the care setting. Written information was also provided for staff who were unable to make the briefing sessions. The briefing sessions are important from an evaluation perspective on two counts:

- They provide an opportunity for one key group of stakeholders (staff) to be included in discussions.

- They enable the evaluator to develop insights into the culture of care that may be present, based on the input of staff to these sessions (this can include low turnout to the sessions).

Conduct of mapping

DCM offers a means to legitimately sit in a setting, make notes and generally have a passive role for a six-hour period. Interesting insights from the conduct of mapping include the tendency for some staff to disappear/avoid the areas where the evaluator is present. This can suggest a number of things. For example, it might suggest discomfort with the process of being observed or a lack of involvement/commitment to the evaluation process. It might alternatively suggest a culture of care where care staff are involved in personal care conducted in private areas (bathrooms and bedrooms), with the remainder of the participant's day spent in communal public areas where little social care is provided.

Staff feedback

Giving staff prompt feedback at the end of an evaluation period can provide reassurance that the evaluator is aware of constraints to care provided. Feedback can recognize difficulties encountered during the care day and give recognition to examples of good care practice, as well as simply thanking staff for their patience with the process.

Formal feedback after having examined the data can be a tricky process for the evaluator. In our experience, staff question the coding frames (often legitimate queries), question the process of observing (is it person-centred?), and question the likelihood of the process making a difference to care practices. We have also found that staff are often willing to embrace the opportunity to set objectives for themselves, for example to try and introduce some form of organized activity each day, to ensure opportunities for people with dementia to go into the garden or for outings into the community.

Impact on mapper

DCM provides an opportunity to observe, from a detached position, the care that people with dementia receive. This may be relatively easy if a mapper comes to the setting with little prior knowledge of or intimacy with the participants who will be observed during the six-hour map. However, if the mapper has previously formed relationships with the participants and has come to know their idiosyncrasies, their patterns of relating with others, particularly with other people with dementia, and their individual ways of expressing distress, the process of mapping might become a painful experience if insensitive care is observed. If patients are left isolated, with their physical or psychological needs going unnoticed, or if interactions with other patients are verging on misunderstandings and conflict while care staff remain oblivious, the mapper may experience increasing discomfort and a decrease in his or her own well-being. This negative impact highlights the need for a support network for mappers in which they can debrief (Brooker 2002) or discuss any emotional difficulties that they encounter in their mapping (Edwards 2005).

During the course of mapping, the mapper may be faced with difficult questions. How does the mapper react in the face of a participant's deteriorating well-being while trying to capture a picture of the setting as it is? When does intervening become interfering? At what stage should one interfere rather than intervene? For example, the mapper, who sees someone in unattended distress and who sees that the care staff have noticed but are not paying attention to this distress, may question whether he or she should interfere and comfort the person or whether he or she should intervene and alert staff to the person's need for help. The mapper can alert a member of staff and hope that the situation will be rectified. Alerting a member of staff and observing and documenting how the situation is handled will add valuable data to the map. However, alerting a member of staff will not always guarantee that the situation will be handled with the sensitivity required to reverse any decline. Indeed the mapper may observe that any intervention by staff may result in further decline. If this occurs, the mapper's duty of care to the participant prevails and he or she must abandon the map and do what he or she can to halt any further decline. The cardinal rule is that, while there may well exist a tension between intervening and interfering, the well-being of those with dementia should always come first. Often, a knowledge of the setting and its ethos of care will determine which course of action is appropriate. A need to interfere is indicative that there is something unsatisfactory with the setting and proving this with quantitative data is unnecessary. Detailed written notes are sufficient and will more than make up for the absence of DCM data.

As a nurse, it is unethical to observe and allow a patient's well-being to deteriorate without intervening in some way. As a nurse/researcher this ethic must also apply. In the hospital ward study the researcher justified all the times she stepped in on the basis that, as a nurse, the well-being of her participants took precedence over research.

Reflections on strengths and limitations of Dementia Care Mapping

We will now reflect on our experiences of the strengths and limitations of DCM.

Strengths

The Audit Commission suggested that the use of DCM to evaluate care can 'greatly enhance the awareness and understanding of staff to improve the care they provide' (2000, p.76). Thus, the evaluator can use the DCM method as a way to disseminate the principles underpinning the DCM method of person-centred care and to encourage staff discussion and reflection on their workplace care practices. However, for this process to occur the evaluator must be aware of what person-centred care means. This concept is the subject of debate at both practitioner and theoretical levels. For example, Packer (2000a) has asked the question 'does person-centred care exist?' and described the challenges facing practitioners in implementing the perceived idealistic goals of person-centred care in resource-scarce situations, and the absence of team work in care settings (Packer 2000b).

From the care home research (Innes 2000) it was clear that staff were open to receiving information through DCM feedback sessions about the lives of those they cared for. For example, in one home the manager commissioned a local artist to work on murals in each wing of the home, the subject of each reflecting the interests of those living there: wildlife and animals. In addition, the corridors were personalized in an attempt to help those who walked around looking for their rooms to locate them more easily. For example, ballet shoes were painted on the wall beside the door of a woman who liked to dance.

Care plans can also be reviewed following a DCM evaluation (Innes 2003b). If an evaluation reveals very little activity, steps can be taken to try and ensure that each individual living in a care home is provided with opportunities to engage in activities that they enjoy: for example art work, reading or gardening. Similarly, if there are certain behaviours that appear excessive, for example distress, then staff can be alerted to this and begin to work through individualized care strategies to address this and improve the care they offer.

DCM can help identify staff training needs and training programmes can be developed to address areas that staff appear to find problematic. However, as Muller-Hergl (2003) points out, organizations using DCM as part of their evaluation and review processes need to be fairly advanced in their learning about dementia and dementia care. If they are not, then small-scale piecemeal initiatives are not likely to succeed. There are, however, accounts of organizations incorporating DCM evaluations into their work culture. For example Scurfield-Walton (2003) describes the strategy her organization adopted in an attempt to address staff development needs and to improve care.

Theoretical reflections on person-centred care for dementia and for gerontological nursing are provided by Brooker (2004) and by McCormack (2004) respectively.

Brooker (2004) suggests that there are four elements that result in person-centred care for people with dementia:

- Valuing people with dementia and those that care for them.

- Treating people as individuals.

- Looking at the world from the perspective of the person with dementia.

- Providing a positive social environment in which the person with dementia can experience relative well-being.

McCormack (2004) concludes that person-centred gerontological nursing (which includes the care of people with dementia) has four aspects:

- being in relation (social relationships)

- being in a social world (biography and relationships)

- being in place (environmental conditions)

- being with self (individual values).

McCormack's conceptual approach is more philosophical than that of Brooker (2004) but both are useful in considering what a DCM evaluation may lead to in terms of developing care practice resulting in person-centred care. McCormack summarizes the person-centred approach as 'the nurse as a facilitator of an individual's personhood' (2004, p.36). He argues that there is a 'need for nurses to move beyond a focus on technical competence and requires nurses to engage in authentic humanistic caring practices that embrace all forms of knowing and acting, in order to promote choice and partnership in care decision-making' (2004, p.36). Thus the very strength of the DCM method, its potential as a catalyst for discussions leading to change, may be blocked by a prevalent culture of care that diminishes personhood. This may result in a clash between the promoted ideal and the reality of providing care for people with dementia.

Limitations
PRACTICAL ISSUES

Carrying out a six-hour map can be a draining experience, particularly if social or environmental conditions are poor. Preparation is the key in order to carry out the full six hours of mapping with consistency and concentration. The mapper must ensure that he or she has sufficient coding sheets, a watch, pencils, an eraser, a pencil sharpener, note paper and the DCM manual. A supply of nutritious food to dip into and plenty of water is also vital, as taking a break is not advisable. It is also helpful if the mapper wears layers of clothing that can be taken off and put on and wears comfortable shoes, as there may be a lot of walking to be done.

If the mapper is mapping alone, as in the case of a PhD student or researcher, there are several issues to consider. The mapper may be mapping in a setting in which those being mapped are scattered about the setting, and engaged in different types of activity. For example, someone may be engaged in conversation in one area while someone else is taking part in a ball game in another area. The lone mapper will be unable to map each person for the full five minutes and will have to decide whether to capture the essence of what each person is doing over a shorter time or to omit one person's BCC for that time frame. Only the mapper can decide what the most appropriate decision is on that particular occasion, but with increasing experience and by seeking advice from more experienced mappers these decisions will become easier.

The lone mapper will also be faced with the issue of the reliability of his or her coding: the degree to which the mapper's choice of coding adheres to the DCM manual and its operational rules. It is recommended that mappers work with at least one other mapper during any DCM evaluation (Surr and Bonde Neilsen 2003). This allows them to check for inter-rater reliability: the extent to which two mappers' maps will be consistent with each other (Woods and Lintern 2003). The lone mapper, who does not have the opportunity of checking his or her reliability, is vulnerable to a subsequent critique of his or her coding so must take other measures to ensure reliability. He or she must take accurate and detailed notes to accompany BCCs and WIB values in order to justify later any coding decision. He or she must seek advice from more experienced mappers if there is doubt about particular codings and he or she must be prepared to change a coding if, with hindsight, it appears inappropriate.

The final issue that the lone mapper has to consider, in the absence of a fellow mapper, is how to debrief, particularly if struggling to cope with a poor environment. Mapping can be a painful experience, especially if, over a period of time, the researcher develops an empathy with his or her participants. The need to remove oneself from their world can be very difficult and can result in feelings of guilt at not being able to engage with them while mapping. One way of resolving guilt at having to temporarily remove oneself from the participants is to engage with them on completion of the map. This will help to re-establish a rapport with them, and may also act as a debriefing session for the participants in which the mapper can discuss aspects of their day with them. The mapper may also gain more insight, from their perspectives, on how their day has gone. While Edwards (2005) calls for a national support network for mappers, at the very least the mapper must seek support from fellow academics, professionals or friends, or in the case of a PhD student, a supervisor or mentor.

LIMITATIONS WITH CODING

DCM has been developed with western concepts of well-being in mind: activity and assertiveness, self-expression and the ability to initiate social contact. The appropriateness of such concepts has been questioned. Kwok (2003) asserts that western notions of well-being are incompatible with

Chinese philosophy. This concern should be borne in mind when mapping a person with dementia whose origins are not western. However, this also raises issues around generalizing BCCs to all people with dementia. For example, Capstick (2003) argues that DCM's interpretation of C (being socially uninvolved, withdrawn) is overly prescriptive and pessimistic and does not allow for the possibility that the person may be in a meditative state. Furthermore, if a person has always been reserved, introverted and content with her own company, it is less likely that he or she will initiate social contact than someone who was sociable and outgoing. But operational rules dictate that certain codes take priority over others, for example A (interacting with others, verbally or otherwise) takes precedence over C. C, being the opposite of activity and occupation, typical of industrialized societies, is given only negative values, implying that this is an undesirable state to be in. As this may not always be the case, there may be times when the mapper finds that he or she is inferring a state of ill-being on a person erroneously. This appears to contradict the person-centred ethos of DCM.

The limitations of DCM were seen most clearly when analysing the video footage from the hospital ward study. There was a vide variety in participants' attendance times at the creative sessions and therefore the length of video footage obtained ranged from 5 to 50 minutes. In DCM terms, some of these time scales are minute and, if analysed following DCM rules, would produce minimal data. One crucial issue emerged from the attempt to analyse the footage using DCM: it does not capture the subtleties of action and interaction. The ability to repeatedly review the video footage allowed the researcher to identify fleeting subtle actions and interactions that seemed to be of importance for the participant, but which, with the application of operational rules, would not have been coded.

For example, during the first time frame of one session, a usually reticent, tense man initiated contact which was mirrored by the care worker who was assisting him at the creative session. There then followed reciprocal smiling and engagement from both parties which, while only lasting 19 seconds, was a significant length of time for this usually isolated man. There followed a few minutes where he watched what she was painting with interest, followed by a short spell during which he replaced the lid of a pastel box and positioned it on the table in work-like fashion.

Within this five-minute time frame three significant events occurred: he initiated and managed to sustain an interaction; he took a sustained interest in the activities of the care worker; and he engaged in work-like activity. However, when using DCM, these subtle yet significant events could not all be coded within the one time frame. In the second time frame he used the paintbrush to write lines of random letters. This event lasted nearly four and a half minutes and involved a combination of creative (E), intellectual (I) and work-like activity (L). Again, following operational rules, the variety of his actions could not be coded. If DCM had been the only method of evaluating the creative sessions, the potential value of creative input, or any other meaningful activity, for a person as isolated as this man was, could have been missed.

On another occasion, a significant but subtle change in demeanour was noted in the video footage of a lady who regularly took part in the creative sessions. She expressed a self-assurance and confidence while painting that was not seen outside of creative sessions. She was clearly engaging in expressive or creative activity (E), but there was also an element of work-like activity (L) as she had been a painter all her life, and there was clearly the emergence and expression of a past self for which there is no BCC.

For an approach that puts person-centredness at its core, it seems that DCM does not provide space for hearing the voice (Capstick 2003) or recognizing self-expression of the person with dementia. These do seem to be critical omissions in the design of this tool. These limitations in approach reflect the thinking when DCM was first developed that the capacity for self-expression is limited in people with dementia. As such, further development of DCM is required in order to do justice to the capacity for self-expression. This is unlikely to occur until DCM 9 or until a 'family of DCM measures' is developed (Brooker 2003). Until then, the mapper's only solution is to use the Positive Events Record to document such instances of self-expression, its facilitation by staff and its significance for the person with dementia.

Kitwood (1997) described in some detail a provisional list of 12 elements of positive person work that are the foundations for the Positive Events Record. For example, he described play, negotiation, recognition, celebration and relaxation which, he argued, will uphold the personhood of people with dementia. These concepts were developed by Kitwood after publication of the seventh edition of the DCM manual (the version we used in our research). In this edition, positive event recording is under-developed and has yet to be operationalized, as evidenced in the fact that only two pages are devoted to it in the manual. Much more work needs to be done in order that positive person work can be documented and evaluated to the same extent as personal detractions.

A tool kit for evaluating dementia care

We found that some staff seemed to find it quite easy to maintain a relatively caring role over the six hours of mapping, but it was more difficult for them to sustain it over the several weeks that the mapper 'hung out' in the ethnographic part of her hospital study. This highlights a limitation of just using DCM to evaluate a setting, but it also highlights the usefulness of linking other methods with DCM in order to develop a fuller picture of the care setting.

In our experience, DCM was not sufficient in itself to evaluate dementia care in long stay care settings. This realization came about as we each struggled with BCC and PE issues and with the application of operational rules. As reflective practitioners and with our increasing sensitivity to the experiences of the people with dementia that we mapped, it became inevitable to want to move beyond the constraints of the framework and to want to take a more holistic approach to evaluating the care that these people received.

We selected additional tools to help establish baseline evidence about care provision and also used additional tools at other specified periods for the duration of the evaluation projects. This has led us to reflect on the need for a 'tool kit' of techniques available to those who take on the role of evaluating long stay dementia care settings. The techniques we have used when evaluating long stay dementia care settings include audit tools to evaluate the care environment; this includes both the physical environment (for example how many rooms are single and have en-suite facilities?) and the staff environment (is there a staff room? what is the rate of staff turnover?). An ethnographic approach in which the evaluator 'hangs out' in the care setting and observes, in a loosely structured way, the daily events in a setting is also useful. Here, the evaluator 'looks, listens and records' (Silverman 2005, p.45) and uses the resultant detailed field notes as further sources of data.

Speaking to people with dementia is a vital part of any evaluation of care (see Chapter 12 for an in-depth discussion of this issue). This can take the form of conversations during ethnographic observation periods or through planned interviews. Similarly, talking to staff about their views and experiences is another way to evaluate long stay care settings. As with people with dementia, this may take the form of structured interviews or conversations during ethnographic observation periods.

While we propose the use of a tool kit when evaluating dementia care, we are not advocating the abandonment of DCM as a useful framework within which to work. DCM gives practitioners and evaluators, particularly those who are new to the person-centred approach, a philosophical and practical starting point for understanding the impact of the social, psychological and physical environment on those with dementia. It serves first as a scaffold to support and reinforce person-centred thinking, but with increasing experience and reflexivity, inevitably it will be seen as one tool among others. We suggest that, in order to grow as reflective practitioners, we must move beyond the constraints of the scaffold and work within the more holistic approach facilitated by a 'tool kit' approach of which DCM is but a part.

The value in a 'tool kit' approach is the opportunity it creates for those undertaking an evaluation of a care setting to select the techniques appropriate for the aspect of care they are planning to evaluate. This enables a range of techniques to be considered and used appropriately, rather than selecting a tool that is in vogue at a particular moment in time.

References

Adams, T. (1996) 'Kitwood's approach to dementia and dementia care: a critical but appreciative review.' *Journal of Advanced Nursing 23*, 948–953.
Audit Commission (2000) *Forget Me Not: Mental Health Services for Older People.* London: The Audit Commission.

Beavis, D. (1998) 'Personal detractions – a personal account.' *Journal of Dementia Care*, July/August, 24–25.

Bradford Dementia Group (1997) *Evaluating Dementia Care: The DCM Method.* Bradford: Bradford Dementia Group.

Brooker, D. (2002) 'Dementia Care Mapping: a look at its past, present and future.' *Journal of Dementia Care*, May/June, 33–36.

Brooker, D. (2003) 'Future challenges for Dementia Care Mapping.' In A. Innes (ed.) *Dementia Care Mapping: Applications Across Cultures.* Baltimore: Health Professions Press.

Brooker, D. (2004) 'What is person-centred care in dementia?' *Reviews in Clinical Gerontology 13*, 215–222.

Brooker, D. (in press) 'Dementia Care Mapping (DCM): a review of the research literature.' *The Gerontologist.*

Brooker, D., Edwards, P. and Benson, S. (eds) (2004) *Dementia Care Mapping: Experience and Insights into Practice.* London: Hawker.

Capstick, A. (2003) 'The theoretical origins of Dementia Care Mapping.' In A. Innes (ed.) *Dementia Care Mapping: Applications Across Cultures.* Baltimore: Health Professions Press.

Dewing, J. (2002) 'From ritual to relationship: a person-centred approach to consent in qualitative research with older people who have dementia.' *Dementia 1*, 2, 157–171.

Edwards, P. (2005) 'Putting Dementia Care Mapping on the map.' *Journal of Dementia Care*, Jan/Feb, 16–17.

Innes, A. (2000) *Changing the Culture of Care: A Systematic Exploration of the Process of Cultural Change in Three Care Settings.* Doctoral thesis, University of Bradford.

Innes, A. (2002a) 'Dementia Care Mapping: a useful tool for social work?' *Practice 14*, 1, 27–38.

Innes, A. (2002b) 'Student-centred learning and person-centred dementia care.' *Education and Ageing 16*, 2, 229–252.

Innes, A. (ed.) (2003a) *Dementia Care Mapping: Applications Across Cultures.* Baltimore: Health Professions Press.

Innes, A. (2003b) 'Using Dementia Care Mapping data for care planning purposes.' In A. Innes (ed.) *Dementia Care Mapping: Applications Across Cultures.* Baltimore: Health Professions Press.

Innes, A. and Surr, C. (2001) 'Measuring the well-being of people with dementia living in formal care settings: the use of Dementia Care Mapping.' *Aging and Mental Health 5*, 3, 258–268.

Kitwood, T. (1997) *Dementia Reconsidered: The Person Comes First.* Buckingham: Open University Press.

Kuhn, D. and Verity, J. (2002) 'Putdowns and uplifts: signs of good or poor dementia care.' *Journal of Dementia Care 10*, 5, 26–27.

Kuhn, D., Fulton, B.R. and Endelmann, P. (2004) 'Factors influencing participation in activities in dementia care settings.' *Alzheimer's Care Quarterly 5*, 3, 144–152.

Kwok, C. (2003) 'Government policy and medical traditions in Hong Kong.' In A. Innes (ed.) *Dementia Care Mapping: Applications Across Cultures.* Baltimore: Health Professions Press.

McCormack, B. (2004) 'Person-centredness in gerontological nursing: an overview of the literature.' *International Journal of Older People Nursing 13*, 31–38.

Muller-Hergl, C. (2003) 'A critical reflection on DCM in Germany.' In A. Innes (ed.) *Dementia Care Mapping: Applications Across Cultures.* Baltimore: Health Professions Press.

Muller-Hergl, C. (2004) 'The role of the "trusted stranger" in DCM feedback.' *Journal of Dementia Care 12*, 2, 18–19.

Packer, T. (2000a) 'Obstacles to person-centred care delivery Part 1: Does person-centred care exist?' *Journal of Dementia Care 8*, 3, 19–21.

Packer, T. (2000b) 'Obstacles to person-centred care delivery Part 3: Pass the hot potato – is this person-centred team work?' *Journal of Dementia Care 8*, 5, 17–19.

Rossi, P.H., Lipsey, M.W. and Freeman, H.E. (2004) *Evaluation: A Systematic Approach.* Thousand Oaks: Sage.

Sabat, S. (2002) 'Surviving manifestations of selfhood in Alzheimer's disease: a case study.' *Dementia 1*, 25–36.

Scurfield-Walton, M. (2003) 'Dementia Care Mapping and staff development.' In A. Innes (ed.) *Dementia Care Mapping: Applications Across Cultures.* Baltimore: Health Professions Press.

Silverman, D. (2005) *Interpreting Qualitative Data: Methods for Analysing Talk, Text and Interaction* (Second edition). London: Sage.

Surr, C. and Bonde Neilsen, E. (2003) 'Inter-rater reliability in Dementia Care Mapping.' *Journal of Dementia Care*, Nov/Dec, 33–35.

Woods, B. and Lintern, T. (2003) 'The reliability and validity of Dementia Care Mapping.' In A. Innes (ed.) *Dementia Care Mapping: Applications Across Cultures.* Baltimore: Health Professions Press.

Chapter 9

Evaluating Long Stay Interventions
Concealment of Medication

Øyvind Kirkevold

This chapter examines some of the issues around administering medication to residents in nursing homes. In most western countries there is an intensive use of medicine among residents in nursing homes. A Swedish study (Kragh 2004) found that two out of three residents in nursing homes were receiving at least ten different medicines, and one out of three was being treated with at least three different kinds of psychotropic drugs. The chapter focuses on the practice of administering medication covertly and examines how this practice may be evaluated.

The staff in nursing homes

In Norway about 20 per cent of the care staff in nursing homes are registered nurses (RN), about 60 per cent are qualified nursing assistants with one or two years of education, and the remaining personnel are assistants without any formal professional qualifications (Eek and Nygård 1999). Studies from other Scandinavian countries, from the US and the UK indicate that these countries have about the same proportion of RNs in nursing homes, or even lower. The frequency of visits from consultant physicians varies between the institutions.

The residents in nursing homes

Residents in nursing homes are very frail and are often in need of extensive help with the most basic care tasks such as dressing, feeding and walking. In addition, the proportion of residents with dementia is quite high. In Norway at least 75 per cent of the residents in nursing homes are people with dementia. One of the main problems in caring for residents with dementia is that many have behavioural and psychiatric symptoms. The high frequency of psychiatric symptoms in dementia is one possible explanation for the high prescription of psychotropic medications in nursing homes. In addition, the residents are older people; in Norway the average age of the residents is about 84 years and in Sweden about 86 years of age.

'Dementia' is a common term for a series of organic diseases characterized by chronic and irreversible impairment in intellectual, emotional and voluntary functioning. The impairment in intellectual functions such as reduced memory and reduced capacity to make decisions means it is sometimes necessary to prescribe life-sustaining medication even if individuals do not explicitly consent. Impairment in emotional functions may result in paranoid ideas and people with dementia may resist the administration of medication because they think those who give them medicine want to hurt or poison them. In later stages of dementia the resident may not understand that they are receiving medication, even if they are told. They feel a lump in their mouth or an uncomfortable taste, and spit it out.

Medications

The use of many different medicines generates several problems, often connected to poly-pharmacies and other pharmacological issues that are beyond the scope of this chapter. Other problems relate to the administration of the medicines. The low proportion of staff qualified to handle medication and the special problems with compliance and dementia, as discussed, make it necessary to evaluate the administration of medication in nursing homes.

In a review of the literature only a few papers describing problems with administration of medicine in nursing homes were found (Barker *et al*. 2002; Kapborg and Svensson 1999; Treloar, Philpot and Beats 2001;

Wright 2002). This literature review highlighted that the evaluation of medication administration is in general a question of *what* medication the residents get compared with what has been prescribed. Thus, the errors found in most cases relate to the wrong medication or the wrong dosage given at the wrong time. These are serious errors and it is important to develop systems to address these types of error. Only two studies were found which focused on *how* the residents get their medicine (Treloar *et al.* 2001; Wright 2002). It is this second issue which is the focus of this chapter.

Is it safe to blend medicine in the residents' food or drink?

Most medication taken orally goes through the digestion tract together with food, thus ordinary medication (where no action has been taken in the production to protect the chemicals from acid or to extend the release of the chemicals) is safe to mix with food or beverages. Medicines that are sublingual, buccal, eneric coated or extended release will all be affected by the act of crushing (Wright 2002). The different national pharmaceutical product compendiums (examples: www.medicines.org.uk; www. felleskatalogen.no; www.fass.se) contain information on each medicine and whether it is unsafe to crush, chew or split. Even though crushing and splitting of pills may be safe, it is a concern because it can lead to inaccurate dosing that may limit the effectiveness of the medication (Fischbach *et al.* 2001).

Administration of medicine in disguise

In 1996 a nurse in England was suspended from her position because she had added sedatives to a resident's tea on instructions from a physician (Kellett 1996). This case created debate, and was a contributing factor in initiating the research done by Treloar and colleagues investigating such practices in the UK (Treloar, Beats and Philpot 2000). This study showed that 71 per cent out of a selection of 35 residential, nursing and hospital units would occasionally medicate their residents without the resident's knowledge. After this revelation regarding the practice of administering medication covertly in Britain the ethics of this practice were debated. One response was to say that this practice is merely an exercise in paternalistic self-righteousness and an invitation to legal disaster (Honkanen 2001). Other responses were more nuanced and asked for guidelines for the covert administration of medication in food and beverages (Treloar *et al.* 2001; Welsh and Deahl 2002).

The strong reaction to this revelation was a surprise because the practice of mixing medicine in the residents' food is well known among staff in nursing homes. In an article in *The Norwegian Nursing Magazine* in 1994 (Carstens 1994) entitled 'Do the residents with dementia know that they were given medicine?' the practice was discussed. Recommendations for how to handle situations where the residents resist medication were given, even though there was no basis in the legislation for such practice. In a report from the Norwegian Health Inspectorate the same year (Aase 1994) the practice of administering medication covertly was mentioned as an example of malpractice in nursing homes. When I have asked nurses working with older people with dementia or other mental health problems, all over Europe, about the practice of giving medicine in disguise, all confirmed that this is a known practice, and some referred to it as quite commonplace.

In 2000, a large nursing home study in Norway was carried out, focusing on the use of restraints, coercive measures and the quality of care in nursing homes (Kirkevold, Sandvik and Engedal 2004). The background for the study was a request from the Department of Health and Social Affairs in 2000. They wanted more knowledge to assess the need for a revision of the legislation regarding the care of persons with reduced capacity.

One of the datasets contained information about whether the medicine given to the residents was hidden in food or not, who decided to use this practice and how it was reported in the residents' records (Kirkevold and Engedal 2005). An in-depth analysis of this dataset evaluated the practice of administering medication covertly. The main reason for the evaluation was the debate in the UK following the study by Treloar and colleagues described above. The data were collected by structured interviews with professional carers of a random sample of 1501 residents in regular nursing homes in 54 municipalities, from all five health regions in Norway.

Of these residents, 1057 lived in regular units and 444 lived in special care units for people with dementia. In addition 425 residents from five teaching nursing homes were included, of whom 305 lived in regular units and 120 lived in special care units. This gave a total of 1926 residents. For each resident, degree of dementia, performance in the activities of daily living, and behavioural disturbance were assessed. Data about ward characteristics, such as size, staffing, and type of ward, were also included. If any drugs had been concealed in the food or beverages during the previous seven days without the resident's knowledge or consent, it was recorded, along with the reason for hiding the drugs. Only recorded drugs given on a regular basis were included in the analysis. Since the practice of giving medicine without the resident's consent is not only ethically questionable, but also is in most cases illegal, all information was given under guarantees of full anonymity. Not only information about the persons who gave the information, but also all information about which nursing home or municipality the information had been collected from, was kept confidential.

Eleven per cent of the residents in regular nursing home units and 17 per cent of the residents in special care units for people with dementia received medicine mixed in their food or beverages at least once during seven days. In 95 per cent of these cases the medicines were routinely mixed in the food or beverages. However, this practice was recorded in the residents' records in only 40 per cent of the cases. The concealment of medicines was most frequently recorded when it was a physician who took the decision to hide the medicine in the residents' foodstuff (57%). Residents who got medicine covertly more often received antiepileptics, antipsychotics and anxiolytics compared to residents who received the medicine openly. In 54 per cent of the cases, 'non-compliance' was the reason given as to why the medicine was given covertly. Non-compliance meant that the resident refused to take the medicine, or spat it out. The second most frequent reason was due to problems with swallowing, 28 per cent. To carry through the necessary medical treatment was also a common reason, 10 per cent. Severe dementia, low function in activities for daily living and aggressive behaviour were the factors most frequently associated with residents who were administered medication covertly.

The arbitrariness in decision making and documentation, and the fact that data were collected from the professional carer, meant that the study accessed information about covert medication that may have been disguised from the physician and head nurse. Thus, those who are responsible do not appear to have taken any action to improve the practice.

The majority of cases in this study involved medicine given in food or beverages as a routine practice. This indicates that the method used did not catch sporadic episodes of covert medication. It is also reasonable to believe that episodes of covert medication that are obviously harmful or which constitute abuse are not reported in this study.

A British study (Macdonald, Roberts and Carpenter 2004) found that in 43 per cent of the nursing homes studied, the practice of administering medication covertly sometimes occurred, but only 4.7 per cent of the residents in the same nursing homes had received medicine covertly. This may indicate that the debate in the UK has reduced the practice of administering medication covertly, or it may be a result of the under-reporting of such practice.

To gain more knowledge about the decision processes leading to the practice of covert medication, more studies are needed. Nevertheless, it would appear that medicines are too often given in disguise to residents who may not want medication, and that it does not necessarily improve the quality of their lives. This raises the question of why particular medications are being prescribed. I will return to this issue later in the chapter but first it is important to address issues of capacity and competence in relation to decisions concerning medication.

Capacity and competence

The terminology around capacity and competence is complex and contentious. There seems to be a general agreement that the terms 'competence' and 'incompetence' refer to a person's legal status, whereas physicians more often talk about mental functioning in terms of the resident's 'capacity' (Post and Whitehouse 1995). However, some prefer to use the terms 'capacity' or 'incapacity' for legal status (Gove and Georges 2001; Jones 2001). Thus, 'capacity' and 'competence' are used synonymously in legal terminology. In cases when a person is incompetent, most West European countries have legal provisions that allow for the appointment of a guardian to handle an adult person's welfare or financial interests (Gove and Georges 2001; Kapp 2001). Separate from this, medical treatment or care without the resident's consent is usually controlled through the mental health legislation. How the decline of functional capacity in different areas relates to 'legal competence' (or 'legal capacity') to make decisions is more complicated and requires an individual assessment for each resident. In most European countries it is forbidden (in long-term care) to give medicine without the resident's consent, but there is a noticeable change in the attitude of the legislation makers. Scotland has the Adults with Incapacity (Scotland) Act 2000 which under special circumstances allows for treatment without the resident's consent (Wilkinson 2001); however, it is doubtful that covert medication is justified by this Act. In Norway similar legislation is expected to pass through Parliament during 2006. In Sweden a committee has been appointed to judge the need for regulations of services for people with dementia who have reduced capacity for autonomous actions.

Autonomy

Autonomy is defined as the capacity to think, decide and act on the basis of rational thought (Harrison 1993; Hillan 1993). It is important to question whether people with dementia are capable of autonomous thought and actions or not. Harrison (1993) concludes that people with dementia are probably capable of autonomous actions in the early stages of the disease, but that they later lose their autonomy. It is obvious that the capacity to make decisions is not reduced to the same degree in the early stages of dementia compared to later in the progression. Wilkinson (2001) has suggested three aspects that should be considered when judging the autonomy of people with dementia. First, a diagnosis of dementia does not automatically mean a judgement of incapacity, as the person may still be able to make a range of decisions. Second, persons with dementia are a heterogeneous group with respect to cognitive capacity and decision-making capacity. Third, an individual's level of understanding can vary according to the nature or complexity of the decision to be taken. In addition it is important to consider the consequences of a decision. Low-risk consequences can offset limits in capacities, whereas high-risk consequences require a more stringent assessment (Post and Whitehouse 1995).

Why evaluate covert medication in nursing homes?

A large proportion of the residents in nursing homes have dementia of severe degree. Considering the discussion of competence and autonomy, and the use of psychotropic drugs for these residents, there is reason to believe that the practice of administering medication covertly is contentious. It is not justifiable to 'treat' people with dementia in long-term care with psychotropic drugs in situations where they themselves do not benefit from the medication. The following discussion focuses on examples where medications may be used to benefit staff in nursing homes or due to pressure from families.

When the practice is undertaken for the benefit of the staff, there is either a severe problem in the 'culture' of care or a serious lack of staff in general, and in particular of qualified staff. For several reasons it would be practical to make the distinction between medication for psychiatric and somatic disorders. It is easier to justify that drugs are mixed in food and beverages to treat a somatic disorder, such as diabetes, heart failure and others, even though such medications do not always benefit the resident. In the United Kingdom Central Council for Nursing, Midwifery and Health Visiting (UKCC) position statement it is stated that the practice of covert medication can be used to protect other residents ('or for safety of others') (UKCC 2006). I feel that this is very problematic. It is obvious that the UKCC advice refers to medications that can be used to control behaviour, to benefit others. This brings us back to the question of for whose benefit the medication is administered. It may be honourable to consider other residents' well-being, and it may be justifiable to treat one resident with chemical restraints to protect other residents, but it may not be so. In a qualitative study concerning nursing staff's attitudes (Malmedal 1999), it was found that sedatives were given to reduce the work burden on the staff. Medication was given because of the staff members' situation. There are also some indications that the families of the residents are less restricted in the practice of giving medicine covertly than nursing staff (Treloar *et al.* 2000). It may be that they are ashamed of their loved ones when they do not behave as before; this argument is then used as a justification for sedation.

The following facts make it crucial to have a continuous monitoring and evaluation of the administration of medicine in nursing homes:

- Residents with moderate or severe dementia (the least competent) are most frequently given medicine in disguise.

- The medication does not always benefit the resident.

- The medicine is often given covertly without the knowledge of the physician who prescribed the medication.

- This is often done in a context with a low proportion of qualified nurses.

- Family members should not be given the responsibility of judging the importance of medication.

Evaluating the administration of medicine in nursing homes

The first step is to admit what is going on. The practice of administering medication covertly has not only been disguised from the residents but also from local and central inspection, as reflected in the low frequency of written documentation of the practice. The quality of written reports in the residents' records is also often found to be poor (Kirkevold 2001). In particular, actions that limit the residents in different ways on a doubtful legal basis seem to be hugely under-reported (Kirkevold and Engedal 2004).

It is the physician and/or nurse who is head of the ward or home that have the responsibility to evaluate practices regarding the administration of medicine on a day-to-day basis. The ability to evaluate how well these routines function will depend on the quality of the written records. One way to improve the documentation is to include information about the residents' capacity to understand what kind of medicine they get and why they get the medicine. Reporting information about the residents' capacity to consent or not consent, how the medicine was administered, and actions that do not follow standard procedure should be mandatory and recorded in the residents' records. In addition the record must also justify that the medication is in the resident's best interest; that all other methods of administration have been unsuccessfully tried; that the doctor who prescribed the medicine had agreed on the method to be used; and that the form of the drug is safe to use covertly (Griffith and Davies 2003). It is important that this information is easy to access for those who inspect and evaluate nursing homes. Information about any deviation from standard routines should always be used in the internal quality assurance programmes in the institutions.

It may be a problem that some of the staff give medicine covertly on their own initiative and may not be interested in reporting it. It might be sleeping pills or tranquillizers on a night shift or other situations where a carer is alone with the residents over a period of time. It is therefore important to be open about these issues. In some cases it may be necessary to carefully follow up staff members who report no problem with administration of medication, where others frequently (or always) experience problems.

Since little is done in the area of administration of medicine regarding covert administration and autonomy, it is necessary to develop and implement registration tools and routines. These would enable daily evaluation of the practice and raise the quality of medicine administration in nursing homes.

How to reduce the practice of mixing drugs in food and beverages

In September 2001 the United Kingdom Central Council for Nursing, Midwifery and Health Visiting (UKCC 2006) published a six-page position statement on covert administration of medicines. This statement was a result of the discussion in the UK described earlier. In this statement the registered nurse is given a great responsibility:

> As a general principle, by disguising medication in food or drink, the resident or client is being led to believe that they are not receiving medication, when in fact they are. The registered nurse, midwife or health visitor will need to be sure that what they are doing is in the best interests of the resident or client, and be accountable for this decision. (p.1)

When it is considered to give medicine without the resident's consent the UKCC summarize as follows:

The UKCC recognises that there may be certain exceptional circumstances in which covert administration may be considered to prevent a resident or client from missing out on essential treatment. In such circumstances and in the absence of informed consent, the following considerations may apply:

- The best interests of the resident or client must be considered at all times.
- The medication must be considered essential for the resident's or client's health and well-being, *or for the safety of others* [my emphasis].
- The decision to administer a medication covertly should not be considered routine, and should be a contingency measure. Any decision to do so must be reached after assessing the care needs of the resident or client individually. It should be resident or client-specific, in order to avoid the ritualised administration of medication in this way.
- There should be broad and open discussion among the multi-professional clinical team and the supporters of the resident or client, and agreement that this approach is required in the circumstances. Those involved should include carers, relatives, advocates, and the multi-disciplinary team (especially the pharmacist). Family involvement in the care process should be positively encouraged.
- The method of administration of the medicines should be agreed with the pharmacist.
- The decision and the action taken, including the names of all parties concerned, should be documented in the care plan and reviewed at appropriate intervals.
- Regular attempts should be made to encourage the resident or client to take their medication. This might best be achieved by giving regular information, explanation and encouragement, preferably by the team member who has the best rapport with the individual.
- There should be a written local policy, taking into account these professional practice guidelines. (UKCC 2006, pp.5–6, reproduced with permission)

Giving clear advice and description of routines for using an illegal practice may create an impression that such practice is legal. The paragraphs above could be used to carry out physical restraints and the locking of doors in the nursing homes or wards. It seems that by labelling such actions as 'medical treatment' it is easier to justify the malpractice compared to a situation when the malpractice is labelled 'caring'. We know that in many cases the administration of medication covertly is done to produce chemical restraints. Medications are used to handle difficult situations that often do not benefit the residents. The use of sedatives may make activities such as bathing, dressing and feeding much easier and limit the need for compulsion. It would, however, be better to use other measures to carry out necessary care tasks than to medicate the residents, if it is done in a gentle and caring way. Most of the situations that are described to justify covert medication could, with better knowledge, routines and resources, be solved without medication or any compulsory measures.

The UKCC guidelines including the above remarks are a good start but it is important to emphasize the role of the physician in long-term care. The prescription of medications is the responsibility of the physician, and the way these medications are to be administered is also included in this responsibility. The role of the physician is critical in the use of medication in a nursing home. A Norwegian study found that physicians with a full-time position in geriatric medicine are less willing to prescribe antipsychotic medications for individuals in a nursing home (Nygaard *et al.* 1994). Schmidt and Svarstad (2002) in a Swedish study found that the quality of communication between nurse and physician had a significant effect on both the use of psychotropic drugs and other problems with poly-pharmacy. Although these studies did not deal with covert medication or administration of medications, they showed that the physician has an important role. It is likely that a combination of more full-time nursing home physicians and a systematic development of good co-operative structures between nurses and physicians will have a positive effect on how medication is being administered, and reduce the use of covert medication. One way to improve the understanding between physicians and nurses would be to train them together (Casey and Smith 1997). With this in mind, the lack of RNs is a concern. When less than 20 per cent of the nursing home personnel are RNs, it could be difficult to achieve appropriate co-operation between nurses and physicians.

The high proportion of carers without any training in nursing homes is a challenge. In addition, qualified nurses need up-to-date knowledge regarding the administration of medicine. In other areas, such as the use of restraint, staff training and information about legislation has reduced the frequency of unwanted practice (Levine, Marchello and Totolos 1995). In most western countries, the legislation does not take into account diminishing capacity following dementia. Thus a revision of the law followed by systematic training programmes for the staff in nursing homes would probably have a positive effect on the quality of administration of medicine.

Concluding remarks

It may seem odd to focus on covert medication when other issues about medication are as problematic. To give sedatives to a resident with dementia who does not understand what he is getting, even when it is given openly, is probably more ethically controversial than mixing diuretics in the food of another resident who may spit it out due to the bad taste. Dementia, aggressive behaviour and poor functioning in ADL are strongly associated with several types of malpractice in nursing homes (Kirkevold and Engedal 2005). The connections are complex. By drawing attention to the practice of covert medication other areas of concern may benefit. The practice of giving medicine in disguise is relatively easy to identify. The responsibility of the physician in prescribing and of the RN in administration is clear, and the problem is quite limited. It should be practicable to implement a project to address the practice of covert medication in long-term wards. Better routines can lead to more co-operation relating to medication and improve situations where the resident does not wish to take medication, especially those where chemical restraints now are used. Staff need a positive contribution from the physician in the form of advice on how better to handle difficult situations where chemical restraints are utilized today. Discussions should take place across professional lines, improving the chances of finding alternative approaches.

References

Aase, K.A. (1994) 'Skremmende bruk av tvang.' *Journalen Sykepleien 82*, 17, 28.

Barker, K.N., Flynn, E.A., Pepper, G.A., Bates, D.W. and Mikeal, R.L. (2002) 'Medication errors observed in 36 health care facilities.' *Archives of Internal Medicine 162*, 16, 1897–1903.

Carstens, N. (1994) 'Vet aldersdemente at de får legemidler.' *Journalen Sykepleien 3*, 28–31.

Casey, N. and Smith, R. (1997) 'Bringing nurses and doctors closer together.' *British Medical Journal 314*, 7081, 617.

Eek, A. and Nygård, A.-M. (1999) *Innsyn og Utsyn – Tilbud til Personer med Demens i Norske Kommuner.* Norway: Nasjonalt Kompetansesenter for Aldersdemens. INFO-Banken.

Fischbach, M.S., Gold, J.L., Lee, M., Dergal, J.M., Litner, G.M. and Rochon, P.A. (2001) 'Pill-splitting in a long-term care facility.' *Canadian Medical Association Journal 164*, 6, 785–786.

Gove, D. and Georges, J. (2001) 'Perspectives on legislation relating to the rights and protection of people with dementia in Europe.' *Aging and Mental Health 5*, 4, 316–321.

Griffith, R. and Davies, R. (2003) 'Accountability and drug administration in community care.' *British Journal of Community Nursing 8*, 2, 65–69.

Harrison, C. (1993) 'Personhood, dementia and the integrity of a life.' *Canadian Journal of Aging 12*, 4, 428–440.

Hillan, E.M. (1993) 'Nursing dementing elderly people: ethical issues.' *Journal of Advanced Nursing 18*, 12, 1889–1894.

Honkanen, L. (2001) 'Point–Counterpoint: is it ethical to give drugs covertly to people with dementia? No: Covert medication is paternalistic.' *Western Journal of Medicine 174*, 4, 229.

Jones, R.G. (2001) 'The law and dementia – issues in England and Wales.' *Aging and Mental Health 5*, 4, 329–334.

Kapborg, I. and Svensson, H. (1999) 'The nurse's role in drug handling within municipal health and medical care.' *Journal of Advanced Nursing 30*, 4, 950–957.

Kapp, M.B. (2001) 'Legal interventions for persons with dementia in the USA: ethical, policy and practical aspects.' *Aging and Mental Health 5*, 4, 312–315.

Kellett, J.M. (1996) 'An ethical dilemma: a nurse is suspended.' *British Medical Journal 313*, 7067, 1249–1250.

Kirkevold, Ø. (2001) *Evaluering av Endring i System for Sykepleiedokumentasjon* (Second edition). Göteborg, Sweden: Nordiska hälsovårdhögskolan.

Kirkevold, Ø. and Engedal, K. (2004) 'A study into the use of restraint in nursing homes in Norway.' *British Journal of Nursing 13*, 15, 902–905.

Kirkevold, Ø. and Engedal, K. (2005) 'Concealment of drugs in food and beverages in nursing homes: cross sectional study.' *British Medical Journal 330*, 7481, 20–22.

Kirkevold, Ø., Sandvik, L. and Engedal, K. (2004) 'Use of constraints and their correlates in Norwegian nursing homes.' *International Journal of Geriatric Psychiatry 19*, 10, 980.

Kragh, A. (2004) '[Two out of three persons living in nursing homes for the elderly are treated with at least ten different drugs. A survey of drug prescriptions in the northeastern part of Skane].' *Lakartidningen 101*, 11, 994–996, 999.

Levine, J.M., Marchello, V. and Totolos, E. (1995) 'Progress toward a restraint-free environment in a large academic nursing facility.' *Journal of the American Geriatric Society 43*, 8, 914–918.

Macdonald, A.J., Roberts, A. and Carpenter, L. (2004) 'De facto imprisonment and covert medication use in general nursing homes for older people in South East England.' *Aging Clinical and Experimental Research 16*, 4, 326–330.

Malmedal, W. (1999) *Sykehjemmets Skyggesider når Beboere i Sykehjem Utsettes for Krenkelser og Overgrep.* Oslo: Kommuneforlaget.

Nygaard, H.A., Brudvik, E., Juvik, O.B., Pedersen, W.E., Rotevatn, T.S. and Vollset, Å. (1994) 'Consumption of psychotropic drugs in nursing home residents: a prospective study in residents permanently admitted to a nursing home.' *International Journal of Geriatric Psychiatry 9*, 10, 387–391.

Post, S.G. and Whitehouse, P.J. (1995) 'Fairhill guidelines on ethics of the care of people with Alzheimer's disease: a clinical summary. Center for Biomedical Ethics, Case Western Reserve University and the Alzheimer's Association.' *Journal of the American Geriatric Society 43*, 12, 1423–1429.

Schmidt, I.K. and Svarstad, B.L. (2002) 'Nurse–physician communication and quality of drug use in Swedish nursing homes.' *Social Science and Medicine 54*, 12, 1767–1777.

Treloar, A., Beats, B. and Philpot, M. (2000) 'A pill in the sandwich: covert medication in food and drink.' *Journal of the Royal Society of Medicine 93*, 8, 408–411.

Treloar, A., Philpot, M. and Beats, B. (2001) 'Concealing medication in residents' food.' *Lancet 357*, 9249, 62–64.

UKCC (2006) *Position statement on the covert administration of medicines – disguising medicine in food and drink.* A UKCC document that has been adopted by the NMC. Available at: www.nmc-uk.org/aFrameDisplay.aspx?DocumentID=69.

Welsh, S. and Deahl, M. (2002) 'Covert medication – ever ethically justifiable?' *Psychiatric Bulletin 26*, 123–126.

Wilkinson, H. (2001) 'Empowerment and decision-making for people with dementia: the use of legal interventions in Scotland.' *Aging and Mental Health 5*, 4, 322–328.

Wright, D. (2002) 'Medication administration in nursing homes.' *Nursing Standard 16*, 42, 33–38.

Chapter 10

Evaluating the Experience of People with Dementia in Decision-Making in Health and Social Care

Jeanne Tyrrell

This chapter examines some of the challenges of evaluating people with dementia's views of their involvement in decision-making in health and social care settings. The ideas discussed have arisen from a community-based study in France in 2003. The aim was to evaluate participants' views of freedom of choice. A framework for assessing the conditions of decision-making between care professionals, family carers and the person with dementia is presented. The results of the evaluation are briefly presented and discussed, having been published in some detail elsewhere (Tyrrell, Genin and Myslinski in press). Some methodological challenges that have emerged from this research experience are identified, many of which are likely to arise in other community-based studies of dementia care. Finally, some suggestions are made for further evaluative research in the area of decision-making in health and social care.

Ageing, dementia and freedom in decision-making

Many authors in the field of gerontology have highlighted the constraints and choices 'imposed' on older people with dementia, and this appears to be a problem in many countries. As a result, their rights and freedom to decide are often limited, especially when individuals become dependent or frail. Browne *et al.* (2002) have observed that older people's freedoms are often overlooked and interfered with by professionals or by family members. Such interference is often justified on the grounds that the older person is 'at risk', and that it is in the interest of that person, or in the interests of others, to restrict his liberty or freedom. This phenomenon has been observed, for example, in institutional care settings (Goldsmith 1996; Kitwood 1997; Tadd, Bayer and Dieppe 2002), or when decisions are made about moving into residential homes (Davies and Nolan 2003).

In France, a Charter of Dependent Elderly Patients' Freedoms and Rights was developed in the 1980s, arising from concerns about the treatment of older users of health and social care services. This document has been revised and widely circulated among professionals and establishments involved in the care of older people (Fondation Nationale de Gérontologie 1989). The charter states that older people maintain their rights and freedoms as citizens, even when frail or dependent; for example, older people have the right to choose where they live, to have access to medico-social care, and to receive clear information about their entitlements. However, recent studies (for example, Leroy, Myslinski and De Galbert 2003; Somme 2003) indicate that freedom of choice is limited, as many older people continue to feel excluded from decision-making about their care arrangements. Somme (2003) reviewed survey data from 3500 older people living in several hundred residential care settings around France. Most residents declared that the decision to move into residential care was made by their families or professionals; only a third had felt actively involved in this decision. In another recent French study, interviews were conducted with older people as they were about to move into residential care (Leroy *et al.* 2003). Most respondents said that it was their family who decided for them about moving to a nursing home, and that they felt resigned to the wishes of their relatives.

The number of older people diagnosed with Alzheimer's disease or other forms of dementia is rising, as the detection of dementia has improved in France (Agence Nationale d'Accréditation et d'Evaluation en Santé 2000). As in other countries, more people are diagnosed at earlier stages of the disease compared with previous decades. Some common assumptions about the abilities of people with dementia have had to be reconsidered, in particular issues of insight, awareness and competence (Clare 2003; Howorth and Saper 2003; Michon, Gargiulo and Rozotte 2003). Nevertheless, as their cognitive functioning is gradually impaired, people with dementia become increasingly dependent on other people for assistance with their activities of daily living. Most day-to-day care for people with dementia is provided informally, within the community; this informal care tends to be provided by family members (usually spouses or children), often on a long-term basis.

In the months and years that follow diagnosis, people with dementia and caregivers face a series of decisions, including choices about services, health and safety, and care arrangements (Wackerbarth 2002). Family carers are recognized as a vulnerable group in need of specific support and advice from professionals, given the progressive nature of dementia, and the fact that caregiving is often an unplanned and long-term engagement (Tyrrell 2004). Clark (1999) has argued that the rights of people with dementia become 'tangled inextricably' with the rights of family care-givers. Those with dementia are frequently accompanied by a caregiver when they are seen in health and social care settings, and people with dementia do not necessarily have the same opinions or priorities as their carers! This may explain why decision-making within the families of people with dementia has attracted so much interest in the ethics literature (see, for example, Baldwin *et al.* 2002; Hughes *et al.* 2002). Apart from the stresses associated with informal caregiving, some carers are reluctant to accept professional help or to seek formal care for their relative (Coudin 2004; Tyrrell 2004). However, the dynamics of working with carers and people with dementia in the community have received limited attention from researchers in France, relative to other developed countries such as England or North America (for example, Adams and Clark 1999; Hasselkus 1988).

To date, most research about autonomous decision-making and dementia has focused on the issue of consent for cognitively impaired par-ticipants in drug trials or medical research protocols. While patient partici-pation is essential for clinical research studies, it is often the carer who decides on behalf of the person with dementia, rather than the person himself (Karlawish 2002; Kim, Karlawish and Caine 2002). Sugarman *et al.* (2001) have drawn attention to the dynamics of decision-making between people with dementia and their proxies in the context of choosing to participate in research trials. Their interviews with proxy respondents indicated that the locus of decision-making was often unclear, so that it was difficult to know to what extent the participant had been involved in deciding to participate in research studies. This 'shifting' of power may also be present in day-to-day decisions. More recently, Hirschmann *et al.* (2004) have suggested that medical decision-making by people with Alzheimer's disease may undergo a transition as the disease progresses: patient-involved decision-making (where the person with dementia is the primary decision-maker) is gradually replaced by shared decision-making, and then caregiver-dominated decision-making occurs when carers have taken over the responsibilities of medical decision-making. However, at the time of this project, no previous studies had examined the opinions of people with dementia concerning their experiences of decision-making in the context of day-to-day care, or their views about their choices.

A model for evaluating freedom of choice in health and social care settings

Evaluating the extent to which decisions are made freely by people with dementia poses multiple challenges. The concept of free choice in health and social care settings is complex and difficult to define clearly. A framework for exploring freedom of choice from the patient's point of view has identified five dimensions underlying freedom of decision-making in medico-social settings (Frossard, Boitard and Jasso-Masqueda 2001). These are:

1. the information made available to the patient or service user

2. the extent to which the patient or service user considers he is being listened to (by the professional)

3. the extent to which he is able to express his opinions about the choices being proposed

4.   the time available to reflect before making a decision

5.   the possibility of being able to change one's mind if the choice is not suitable.

These five dimensions can be evaluated using a semi-structured interview, aimed at reviewing the conditions under which a real-life decision has been made. The semi-structured interview includes introductory comments about the context of the study, followed by a series of questions which examine the five dimensions of decision-making. Participants are encouraged to speak freely about their experiences as they respond to the questions, and are prompted by the interviewer to indicate to what extent they were informed, to what extent they had been free to express their views before making their decision and so on. These five criteria are not exhaustive, but they provide a structured way of evaluating the choice processes of people with dementia in health and social care. This approach is applicable to different groups of service users and/or their carers.

Challenges in evaluating freedom of choice in the context of dementia care

Studying freedom of choice and decision-making by people with dementia presents a number of potential difficulties, which may explain why research into these processes is limited. First, cognitive impairment has often been a criterion for *excluding* people with dementia from studies of user satisfaction or those requiring participants' opinions in gerontology research studies. The extent and nature of cognitive decline is highly variable between individuals diagnosed with dementia, even within the early stages of illness. Memory impairment can affect the recall of recent events, which can reduce the richness and reliability of self-report data. Also, there are often uncertainties about the extent to which an individual person's judgement and competence are affected, as well as the degree of insight into his condition (Hirschmann *et al.* 2004; Howorth and Saper 2003). Furthermore, dementia-related communication problems can limit the extent to which participants can talk about their experiences (Santo Pietro and Ostuni 1997).

Nevertheless, as the diagnosis of dementia is being made earlier than in previous decades, health and social care professionals are increasingly encouraged to involve the person with dementia as much as possible in decision-making and discussions about their care. American and British studies have indicated that people in the 'early' and 'moderate' stages of dementia are often capable of expressing meaningful opinions about the quality of care or their quality of life (for example, Brod *et al.* 1999; Mozley *et al.* 1999). Furthermore, Feinberg and Whitlach (2001) have demonstrated that cognitively impaired older participants can give consistent responses to questions concerning their preferences, choices and day-to-day involvement in decision-making.

This chapter draws on the French 'Freedom of Choice' study, the aim of which was to evaluate the conditions of decision-making with people diagnosed with dementia, in order to understand to what degree they had been involved in making choices about their care arrangements. No previous studies exploring this specific issue directly with people with dementia had been found in the international literature. An overview of the methods and main results of the study will be presented briefly here before discussing the methodological challenges that arise when including the views of people with dementia in evaluations. A full account of the study is presented elsewhere (Tyrrell *et al.* in press).

Overview of the 'Freedom of Choice' study

As the study wished to explore people with dementia's experiences of decision-making in health and social care, participants were recruited with the assistance of a network of community-based local psychologists and psychosocial services in Grenoble, France. The criteria for inclusion were that the person (a) had been diagnosed with dementia; (b) was capable of communicating verbally in an interview situation; and (c) had an identified primary caregiver who was available to be interviewed. Letters were sent to ten centres (who had previously agreed to assist with recruitment) detailing the purpose of the study and the profile of people required for inclusion in the study. Each centre then forwarded letters to the designated primary caregivers of such people to explain the purpose of the study and to inform both the older person with dementia and his caregiver that they were invited to participate on a voluntary and confidential basis. Those who wished to participate sent a pre-addressed stamped envelope to the research centre, and a suitable interview time was then arranged by telephone.

Freedom of choice was explored using a semi-structured interview, based on the 'freedom of choice' interview schedule (Frossard *et al.* 2001).[1] Participants were asked to think of a recent situation where they had had to make a choice concerning their health or social care. They were then asked to indicate on a rating scale whether they had been informed adequately; whether they had been listened to; whether they had been able to express their opinion about the options proposed; and whether they had had time to reflect on their choice before making a decision, and to what extent they could change their minds if their decision did not suit them.

Interviews were conducted with 21 pairs of participants (21 people with dementia and their 21 primary carers). The 21 people with dementia were aged between 74 and 91 years, with an average age of 84 years. There were five men and 16 women, all in the early stages of dementia; nevertheless, they were all able to participate in the interview and give meaningful responses. Six were living alone, seven were living with a spouse or relative, and eight had recently been admitted to residential care. The 21 caregivers were aged between 42 and 85 years, with an average age of 62 years. The relationship with the person with dementia varied: 14 were daughters, six were sons, and one was the husband. The first stage of the interview was conducted jointly with the person with dementia and his caregiver in the same room, so that the participant could nominate a recent situation where a decision regarding his care had been made. Each party was then interviewed separately to ensure that independent responses were collected concerning their views of how this choice had been made.

Three types of choices were mentioned in the 21 interviews: the decision to accept help at home (eight cases), the decision to attend a day centre (five cases), and the decision to move into residential care (eight

---

1   An English translation of the interview schedule developed specifically for the dementia care study is published in Tyrrell *et al.* (in press).

cases). Their replies to the five questions about decision-making indicated some of the problems that they had encountered.

The first question examined to what extent participants felt that they had been informed before making their choice. Only four participants felt that they had been well informed about their options, nine said that they were only partially informed and eight said that they were not at all informed. Participants were then asked if they had felt that they were listened to as they were making their decisions. Eight people felt that they had been listened to, eight felt that they had only been partially heard, and five said that they had not been listened to at all. Some people specified that the feeling of not being fully listened to also related to their families and not just professionals. The third issue concerned the opportunity to express opinions about the choices available. The most frequent reply (nine cases) was that the person with dementia had not been able to express their views at all. Six people had fully expressed their views, and six felt that they had only partially expressed their opinions.

Participants were then asked if they had had time for reflection before making their decision. The most frequent reply (13/21 people) was that the choice was made without any time for reflection. Seven participants said they had some time to reflect, but that it was insufficient. Only one person felt that their decision had been taken with adequate time to reflect on their options. Finally, participants were asked about their satisfaction with the decision that had been made, and the possibility of changing one's mind where the decision was unsatisfactory. Eight people felt that their choice was satisfactory, and that they did not wish to change their decision. One person was only partially satisfied with her choice, but felt that she could modify it if she wished. Over half the participants (12 cases) felt that the choice was difficult or impossible to modify; in seven of these cases, the choice concerned entering residential care.

Caregivers' views of decision-making

The first question examined the extent to which carers felt that they had been informed before making their choice. Seven carers felt that they had been very well informed about the options; ten were partially informed; four were not at all informed.

Carers were then asked if they had felt they were listened to, as they were making their decisions. Most carers (13/21) felt that they had been very well listened to by the professionals, although eight felt that they had only been partially heard. In contrast with the older participants, none of the carers felt that they had not been listened to. The third issue concerned the opportunity to express opinions about the choices available. Most carers (15/21 respondents) felt that they had been able to express themselves completely (in contrast to the experiences of the people with dementia). Four carers said that they had only been able to partially express their opinions, and two carers felt that they hadn't had the opportunity to express their opinions at all. Carers were then asked if they had had time for reflection before making the decision. The majority of carers felt that they had had enough time to reflect on the decision (16 cases); this contrasts sharply with the replies of those people with dementia. Four carers said they had some time to reflect, but that it was insufficient. Only one carer felt that the decision had been made without adequate time to consider the options.

Finally, participants were asked about their satisfaction with the decision that had been made, and the possibility of changing one's mind where the decision was unsatisfactory. Nine carers felt that the choice was satisfactory, and that they did not wish to change it. Three carers were partially satisfied with the decision, but felt that it could be modified or reversed. Nine carers felt that the decision once made was difficult to modify or reverse.

People with dementia and their carers' views of decision-making

This study indicates that it is possible to assess views of decision-making with older people who are cognitively impaired, although the modest sample size limits any generalizations. It was not clear at the beginning of the project whether it would be possible to conduct this type of interview with this user group, and if they would be able to recall clearly recent situations of choice. Indeed, before beginning data collection, several experienced clinical colleagues expressed doubts about the feasibility of conducting this type of study with people who had been diagnosed with dementia. However, all 21 participants with dementia were able to complete the interview, and to offer meaningful replies to the questions. Their demographic profile and those of their carers reflected national trends in France, where most people with dementia are older, and most informal carers are female family members.

Overall, the replies of participants to the questions indicate that their decisions had often been made under several constraints (such as inadequate information or lack of time), although carers tended to be more satisfied with the conditions of decision-making. People with dementia were more likely than carers to report that they were not listened to, and that they had not had the opportunity to express their opinions. They were less satisfied than carers with the information provided and with the time available to reflect before making their decision. This may indicate that professionals are more successful at communicating with carers than with service users when choices are being discussed about care arrangements, or that people with dementia are overlooked during negotiations about their future (see Adams and Gardiner 2005; Bender 2003).

Carers and people with dementia had similar views on the fifth dimension (the degree to which a decision can be reversed or modified if necessary), relative to the other dimensions of choice, which are perhaps more subjective. Although over one third of the participants felt that their decision had suited them, many people felt that the choice once made was irreversible, or very difficult to modify. These situations often related to moving into residential care, a decision that is, in reality, often very difficult to change. The implications of these findings for research, education and professional practice have been discussed in some detail elsewhere (Tyrrell *et al.* in press); the remainder of this chapter focuses on some of the methodological issues that arose in conducting this investigation, issues that are likely to arise in other evaluative studies.

Methodological challenges in evaluating the experiences of people with dementia

Several methodological problems arose during this evaluation. Challenges included accessing and recruiting participants, as well as preparing and adapting an interview schedule for people with cognitive impairment (and their carers). Some of these issues are likely to arise in other community-based studies of health and social care for people with dementia.

First, there were considerable difficulties recruiting people with dementia to study their experiences of decision-making; both the target population and the time frame of the study had to be extended in order to have a reasonable sample size. Only 12 interviews were possible from the initial list of 50 potential participants, and a second wave of recruitment was necessary, which was only partially successful. From a total target group of 103 families, 21 pairs of interviews were conducted, a participation rate of about 20 per cent. Some of the difficulties encountered in accessing participants are common to community-based studies with psychiatric patients or older people. The low rate of participation was due to non-responses, refusals, time constraints, illness, unforeseen hospitalizations, and even death. The fact that it was usually carers who determined whether or not the interviews went ahead (and not the person with dementia) is common to other studies with this user group. However, it introduced an important bias into the evaluation, as the majority of people invited to participate did not do so. It seems likely that participants had *higher* levels of freedom than the average person with dementia, given that most in the target group did not have the possibility of expressing their views.

Primary caregivers are frequently asked to give approval or consent for the participation of those they care for in the field of dementia research; this question of consent-by-proxy is an ongoing and controversial issue (see, for example, Bravo, Pâquet and Dubois 2003; Vass *et al.* 2003). Furthermore, previous experiences of recruiting caregivers for studies of carer stress and dementia (Tyrrell 2004) have shown that many caregivers themselves are reluctant to participate in research interviews. This is sometimes because (a) they find it emotionally draining or difficult to reflect on their day-to-day life as caregivers; or (b) they cannot free themselves from the responsibility of caring for their relative to spend an hour being interviewed; it appears that the caregivers who feel most overwhelmed may be less likely to make themselves available for research studies.

Nevertheless, the difficulties experienced with accessing this population is a potential barrier for other studies. Carers act as gatekeepers between evaluators and people with dementia, a phenomenon familiar to those involved in drug trials and clinical research studies. For this reason, I suggest that more attention should be paid to identifying the factors affecting carers' willingness to allow their relatives with dementia to participate in community-based research. People with dementia represent a growing population who are likely to be the focus of different types of studies in the future, and it is not clear to what extent the difficult access is due to carer concerns about participant well-being, time constraints, an unwillingness to reflect on certain aspects of care, or other reasons.

Another source of potential bias in this evaluation arose in the recruitment stage. Local professional colleagues were asked to identify people who they considered to be eligible participants, having provided them with the three inclusion criteria for this study. However, as the evaluation was examining users' experiences of decision-making in health and social care, it is possible that people with dementia or carers who, for whatever reasons, had difficulties working with professionals may have been excluded as unsuitable. Therefore, it is possible that participants may have had more positive views of their experiences of making decisions about health or social care issues than the average user of these services. It is difficult to know how to overcome this type of bias, as research with service users often requires indirect recruitment, where professionals are requested to assist in the identification of suitable participants by applying the researchers' inclusion criteria to their caseload. There is a risk of under-representation of people who are dissatisfied with their experiences of health or social care arrangements.

An unforeseen issue concerns the clinical evaluation of people for inclusion in community-based studies. In health care research, investigators are usually required to indicate to what extent the patient-participants are affected by their illness, for example if they are in the early or late stages of dementia. This information is not easily available in community-based

studies, in contrast with clinic-based studies, where recent assessment data
(neurological evaluations, for example) are often routinely available. Most
people with dementia live at home, rather than in institutional settings. It is
not feasible (nor, some would argue, desirable) to assess or test participants
in their homes prior to interviewing them. This introduces an important
question of how to describe the participants' stage(s) of dementia. Recent
assessment data about illness severity may be available indirectly from
recent hospital admissions, memory clinic assessments or family doctors,
but this was not the case for most of the participants. As explained in a
recent article (Tyrrell *et al.* in press), carer-rated instruments exist which
indicate how well the person is able to function in daily life, but these evaluation tools are not always a reliable indicator of illness severity. This issue
is rarely discussed in the literature, but will remain a challenge in the future
as efforts are made to evaluate community-based dementia care in other
countries. Such studies will need to indicate clearly the clinical status of
participants with dementia-type illness, given the enormous variations in
personal abilities within and between stages of dementia.

The positive experience of interviewing people with dementia
confirms the findings of some other authors (for example, Feinberg and
Whitlach 2001; Mozley *et al.* 1999) that a meaningful *dialogue* is often
possible in the early stages of dementia. This required additional time,
skills and efforts from the evaluators to facilitate the expression of views
(see Chapter 12 for further discussion of this issue). The team member
who conducted the interviews had previous experience in doing interviews for dementia-related studies and undertook training and ongoing
supervision to ensure that interviews were conducted in a way that would
facilitate the expression of opinions and views. Considerable time was
spent studying and revising the original interview schedule to simplify the
language and preparing alternative ways of explaining the questions in
case carers and people with dementia were unclear about what was being
asked. The anticipated abandoning of some interviews, when the questions might be too difficult, did not occur.

In the last decade, more information has been published about communication difficulties associated with dementia (Innes and Capstick 2001;
Powell, Hale and Bayer 1995) and guidelines are available to facilitate

interviews (for example, McKillop and Wilkinson 2004; Santo Pietro and Ostuni 1997). This literature is essential background reading when embarking on studies similar to this one, where interviewing is a key method of data collection. Individuals with dementia experience many difficulties as a result of their illness, including word-finding difficulties, inattention, or slowed processing of speech, which create barriers when communicating with others. Researchers need to be familiar with the potential difficulties and handicaps which may arise as dementia progresses. Furthermore, most people with dementia are over 70 years of age, and may be experiencing additional health problems (such as fatigue) or age-related sensory deficits including hearing loss or visual impairment. Evaluators who are aware of these potential problems and who are trained to facilitate communication with this user group are in a stronger position to establish a good rapport, and to gather reliable data through interviews. These inter-personal skills are an important consideration when recruiting personnel to conduct evaluative studies about dementia care.

Future directions for research into decision-making

At the time of this investigation (2003) there were very few published studies in the field of dementia care which aimed to evaluate specifically people with dementia's experiences of decision-making. It seems likely that more evaluative studies will be required in related areas, such as measuring service user satisfaction, preferences and priorities, and quality of care. The extent to which people with dementia feel involved in decision-making is a promising research theme, given the growing interest in autonomy in the health and social care literature. Nevertheless, the preliminary work raised more questions than it answered. Several suggestions are offered for developing research into the experiences of people with dementia, and widening the methodologies from those employed in this initial study.

This study of participants' experiences was conducted retrospectively, and was limited to a subgroup of people at the early stages of dementia who were capable of participating in an interview and expressing their views about the different stages of decision-making. Retrospective questioning about how a decision was made is less accurate than studying the process of decision-making as it is happening. Aside from the impact of dementia-related memory problems on the person, carers are likely to have some difficulty recalling accurately the specifics of a situation several weeks later. Ideally, the process of decision-making should be studied as it unfolds, but it is unlikely that people with dementia, carers and professionals would welcome additional questions (or observers) at a time when they are considering changes in care arrangements. However, short structured interviews might be possible in the days following the taking of a decision in order to reduce errors or omissions introduced by delayed recall.

From a methodological point of view, the exploration of decision-making was restricted to the five dimensions within the interview schedule. These dimensions are not exhaustive, although they provided a theoretical framework and a pragmatic starting point for the study. The interview data provided preliminary indications about the conditions of decision-making, rather than in-depth knowledge of the circumstances surrounding the choices made. The responses to these five dimensions raise further questions about the extent to which decisions are freely made by people with dementia (and their carers) when accepting professional help at home, or engaging with day care or residential care services. For example, when respondents indicated that they were only partially satisfied with the information received, it is not clear which elements of information had been satisfactory or unsatisfactory. Further studies are required to explore to what extent the information offered is relevant, detailed or clearly explained; these criteria are likely to vary from one person to another, even in the same type of decision-making situation (for example, moving into residential care). Qualitative approaches are required to help answer these questions. Another improvement on the design discussed above would be to target people with dementia according to the types of decision they had made recently, rather than requiring them to nominate a situation of choice at the beginning of the evaluation interview. More background information about the circumstances leading to and influencing the decision would be useful (for example, to what extent did critical incidents or carer stress influence the decision to seek outside help at home, or day care for the person with dementia). Such refinements to the evaluation design would result in a more focused evaluation; the data obtained from this type of study would allow the formulation of more specific recommendations for improving professional support for people with dementia and their carers.

This study did not include the views of the professionals who had been involved with people with dementia and carers when they were making their decisions. Their opinions would have added to our understanding about the conditions of decision-making in the 21 situations. A recurrent theme in the informal verbal feedback from professional colleagues is the lack of alternatives that are available for them to propose to service users. In other words, people with dementia and their carers are often confronted with a restricted palette of 'choices' (often just two possibilities) when problems with home care arrangements require new decisions to be made. Professionals are unable to offer a wider range of choices because of budgetary restrictions or limitations in service developments. A commonly cited example is where a person is faced with the decision to move from home care to residential care. The timing of this decision is often determined by the availability of residential care places, and these are scarce in some areas. Ideally, a person with dementia and his family should be able to visit several nursing homes and 'choose' the most suitable, but this rarely occurs in reality.

It was clear from the interview data that some participants had more positive experiences of decision-making than others, feeling that they had been freer to choose what care arrangements suited them. However, the extent to which staff training might have had an impact on the participants' experience of decision-making was not explored. Professionals trained to recognize and to respect the rights and feelings of people with dementia might be able to foster a sense of being involved in decision-making in such people. Given the increasing interest in developing person-centred dementia care, future evaluative studies might examine the extent to which training programmes for staff can improve people with dementia's involvement in making decisions about their care.

Conclusion

This chapter gives some encouraging indications about the feasibility of interviewing people with dementia about their involvement in decision-making, an issue which is receiving more attention from researchers and evaluators as the diagnosis of dementia has improved in recent years. Some people with dementia feel that their opinions are overlooked, and it appears that their rights to information and free expression are fragile. The data gathered highlight some problems experienced with decision-making and the freedom to choose how to manage care arrangements. As this chapter has explained, the evaluation of people with dementia's experiences of decision-making presents many methodological challenges, some of which are likely to arise in other countries and care settings. However, the inclusion of people's views is an essential element when evaluating their experiences, rather than relying on the views of proxy-respondents. The methodological challenges considered here may help evaluators as they reflect on how to improve the evaluation of dementia care and include the viewpoints of people with dementia.

References

Adams, T. and Clark, C. (1999) *Dementia Care: Developing Partnerships in Practice.* London: Baillière Tindall.

Adams, T. and Gardiner, P. (2005) 'Communication and interaction within dementia care triads: developing a theory for relationship-centred care.' *Dementia 4,* 2, 185–205.

Agence Nationale d'Accréditation et d'Evaluation en Santé (ANAES) (2000) *Recommandations pour le Diagnostic de la Maladie d'Alzheimer.* Paris: ANAES.

Baldwin, C., Hughes, J., Hope, T., Jacoby, R. and Ziebland, S. (2002) 'Ethics and dementia: mapping the literature by bibliometric analysis.' *International Journal of Geriatric Psychiatry 18,* 41–54.

Bender, M. (2003) *Explorations in Dementia.* London: Jessica Kingsley Publishers.

Bravo, G., Pâquet, M. and Dubois, M. (2003) 'Opinions regarding who should consent to research on behalf of an older adult suffering from dementia.' *Dementia 2,* 1, 49–65.

Brod, M., Stewart, A., Sands, L. and Walton, P. (1999) 'Conceptualisation and measurement of quality of life in dementia: the dementia quality of life instrument.' *The Gerontologist 39,* 1, 25–35.

Browne, A., Blake, M., Donnelly, M. and Herbert, D. (2002) 'On liberty for the old.' *Canadian Journal of Ageing 21,* 2, 283–293.

Clare, L. (2003) 'Managing threats to self: awareness in early stage Alzheimer's disease.' *Social Science and Medicine 57,* 1017–1029.

Clark, C. (1999) 'Professional practice with people with dementia and their family carers: help or hindrance?' In T. Adams and C. Clark (eds) *Dementia Care: Developing Partnerships in Practice*. London: Baillière Tindall. pp.280–304.

Coudin, G. (2004) 'La réticence des aidants familiaux à recourir aux services gérontologiques: une approche psychosociale.' *Psychologie et Neuropsychologie du Vieillissement 2*, 4, 285–296.

Davies, S. and Nolan, M. (2003) '"Making the best of things": relatives' experiences of decisions about care-home entry.' *Ageing and Society 23*, 429–450.

Feinberg, L.F. and Whitlach, C.J. (2001) 'Are persons with cognitive impairment able to state consistent choices?' *The Gerontologist 41*, 3, 374–382.

Fondation Nationale de Gérontologie (1989) *Charte des droits et libertés des personnes âgées dépendantes*. Paris: FNG. (Document available in English on www.fng.fr.)

Frossard, M., Boitard, A. and Jasso-Masqueda, G. (2001) *L'évaluation des Coordonnations Gérontologiques*. Grenoble: Fondation de France-CPDG.

Goldsmith, M. (1996) *Hearing the Voice of People with Dementia*. London: Jessica Kingsley Publishers.

Hasselkus, B. (1988) 'Meaning in family caregiving: perspectives on caregiver/ professional relationships.' *The Gerontologist 28*, 686–691.

Hirschmann, K., Xie, S., Feudtner, C. and Karlawish, J. (2004) 'How does an Alzheimer's disease patient's role in medical decision-making change over time?' *Journal of Geriatric Psychiatry and Neurology 17*, 2, 55–60.

Howorth, P. and Saper, J. (2003) 'The dimensions of insight in people with dementia.' *Aging and Mental Health 7*, 2, 113–122.

Hughes, J.C., Hope, T., Savulescu, J. and Ziebland, S. (2002) 'Carers, ethics and dementia: a survey and review of the literature.' *International Journal of Geriatric Psychiatry 17*, 35–40.

Innes, A. and Capstick, A. (2001) 'Communication and personhood.' In C. Cantley (ed.) *A Handbook of Dementia Care*. Buckingham: Open University Press. pp.135–145.

Karlawish, J. (2002) 'Les décisions de patients et de leurs aidants concernant la recherche et le traitement de la maladie d'Alzheimer.' In S. Andrieu and J-P. Aquino (eds) *Les Aidants Familiaux et Professionnels: du Constat à l'action*. Paris: Serdi. pp.157–162.

Kim, S., Karlawish, J. and Caine, E. (2002) 'Current state of research on decision-making competence of cognitively impaired elderly persons.' *American Journal of Geriatric Psychiatry 10*, 151–165.

Kitwood, T. (1997) *Dementia Reconsidered: The Person Comes First*. Buckingham: Open University Press.

Leroy, S., Myslinski, M. and De Galbert, A. (2003) 'Représentations préalables de l'entrée en institution pour la personne âgée et sa famille.' *Gérontologie 125*, 35–41.

McKillop, J. and Wilkinson, H. (2004) 'Make it easy on yourself: advice to researchers from someone with dementia on being interviewed.' *Dementia 3*, 2, 117–125.

Michon, A., Gargiulo, M. and Rozotte, C. (2003) 'Qu'est ce que la démence? La démence vue par le patient.' *Psychologie et Neuropsychologie du Vieillissement 1*, 1, 7–13.

Mozley, C., Huxley, P., Sutcliffe, C., Bagley, H., Burns, A., Challis, D. and Cordingley, L. (1999) '"Not knowing where I am doesn't mean I don't know what I like": cognitive impairment and quality of life responses in elderly people.' *International Journal of Geriatric Psychiatry 14*, 776–783.

Powell, J., Hale, M. and Bayer, A. (1995) 'Symptoms of communication breakdown in dementia: carers' perceptions.' *European Journal of Disorders of Communication 30,* 65–75.

Santo Pietro, M.J. and Ostuni, E. (1997) *Successful Communication with Alzheimer's Disease Patients: An In-service Manual.* Boston: Butterworth-Heinemann.

Somme, D. (2003) 'Participation et choix des résidents dans le processus d'entrée en institution.' *Dossiers Solidarité et Santé 1,* 35–47.

Sugarman, J., Cain, C., Wallace, R. and Welsh-Bohmer, K. (2001) 'How proxies make decisions about research for patients with Alzheimer's disease.' *Journal of American Geriatrics Society 49,* 1110–1119.

Tadd, W., Bayer, T. and Dieppe, P. (2002) 'Dignity in health care: reality or rhetoric?' *Reviews in Clinical Gerontology 12,* 1–4.

Tyrrell, J. (2004) 'L'épuisement des aidants: facteurs de risque et réponses théra-peutiques.' In J. Gaucher, G. Ribes and T. Darnaud (eds) *Alzheimer et l'aide aux Aidants: Une Nécessaire Question Éthique.* Lyon: Editions Chronique Sociale. pp.48–59.

Tyrrell, J., Genin, N. and Myslinski, M. (in press) 'Freedom of choice and decision making in health and social care: views of older patients with early stage dementia and their carers.' *Dementia.*

Vass, A., Minardi, H., Ward, R., Aggarwal, N., Garfield, C. and Cybyk, B. (2003) 'Research into communication patterns and consequences for effective care of people with Alzheimer's and their carers.' *Dementia 2,* 1, 21–48.

Wackerbarth, S. (2002) 'The Alzheimer's family caregiver as decision-maker: a typology of decision styles.' *Journal of Applied Gerontology 21,* 3, 314–332.

PART THREE

Future Challenges in
Evaluating Dementia Care

Chapter 11

Ethics, Evaluation and Dementia

Julie Christie

The person with dementia is subject to increasing dependence on others and an impaired ability to interpret the physical and social world (Martin and Post 1992, p.55). As a result any research or evaluation process that involves a person with dementia is subject to stringent ethical constraints and safeguards. Ethics can be described as constructed norms of internal consistency regarding what is right and wrong (Banks 2001; Osborne 1998). In essence, ethics is a systematic reasoning of how we ought to act. This reasoning is guided by a variety of factors including our internal morals and values, the expectations of wider society and the professional codes of ethics that govern professional practice. Ethical issues refer to the rights of the individual or others and also include wider societal issues (Banks 2001). Ethical decisions include dilemmas as to what you should do as well as what you should not. The range of ethical dilemmas that might be encountered in an evaluation involving a person with dementia are many and varied (Adams and Clarke 1999; Bartlett and Martin 2002). This chapter aims to explore the challenges in addressing the ethical implications of evaluation in dementia care. It will begin by considering the relevance of ethics in dementia practice. It will then proceed to consider the process of evaluation. There will be a discussion about demonstrating accountability to the evaluation participants and consideration given to addressing the issues that arise in the participation of people with dementia in evaluation and research. Throughout this chapter the main points of the discussion will be highlighted as a suggested guide to good practice in this area.

Ethical practice and dementia

The question at the heart of ethical debate when working with people who have dementia is one of personhood: 'Is there a person locked away in the midst of the illness?' (Goldsmith 1999, p.83). Goldsmith believes that the answer to this offers society a reflective opportunity that is not always welcome. Does society consider people who have dementia to be 'non-persons' because they are unable to take moral responsibility for their own choices (Cox *et al.* 1998; Downie and Telfer 1980)? Do we consider people with dementia as less than human?

If we refer to the predominant medical model of dementia, person-hood gradually diminishes and is eventually lost (Goldsmith 1996). Dementia is described in terms of increasing cognitive losses and the 'un-becoming of self' with little reference to the person, their emotional needs or feelings (Fontana and Smith 1989, p.1; Kitwood 1997). A school of thought has however evolved whereby the *label* 'dementia' is considered to be the barrier to inclusion and communication (Kitwood 1996). It argues that the older person with dementia confirms societal expectations of the sick role. Denying our identification with people who have dementia is a means of protecting ourselves from the potential indignities of old age and ill health (Harding and Palfrey 1997). The social disability model of dementia challenges the biomedical approach. It argues that medical explanations of dementia and dependence do not take into account 'the person' and the wider concepts of independence such as decision-making, choice and power (Hill 1999). There has therefore been a growing interest in listening to individual accounts of living with dementia (Davis 1989; Friel McGowan 1993). Seeking the opinion of people who have dementia as the *focus* of research or evaluation however remains relatively rare (Pratt 2002; Robinson 2002).

The starting point of ethical practice in evaluation is the recognition that the person with dementia is not an object for study but a person with views and opinions. Robinson (2002, p.104), speaking as a person with dementia, reminds us that 'It doesn't follow that as soon as you are diagnosed you immediately become incapable of communicating' and asks the question 'Why shouldn't I be included?'

The question is not should the person with dementia be involved but *how* we can make this possible. The skill therefore lies in including the individual with respect, beneficence and integrity (Mark 1996).

The 'Living Well into Old Age' report prepared by the King's Fund Centre (1986) identifies the principles that should be applied when working with people who have dementia. The report clearly states that people with dementia have the same human value as anyone else and the same rights as other citizens. The principle of safeguarding the rights and quality of life of the individual and their family is central to ethical practice. Wilkinson (2002, p.19) advises that enabling the inclusion and participation of people with dementia does however require complex and sensitive consideration before beginning. The values framework designed by Cox *et al.* (1998, p.23) provides a structure for that consideration by identifying five core values that apply to working with people who have dementia. These are:

- maximizing personal control
- enabling choice
- respecting dignity
- preserving continuity
- promoting equity.

The questions outlined in Box 11.1 should be addressed as part of the evaluation planning with reference to these stated values.

Questions about the evaluation

The initial questions about the evaluation are generic and refer to good working practice in undertaking any evaluation or research process. Although not specific to people who have dementia it is worth stating that there are no shortcuts in ensuring ethical practice no matter the client group. Most people are clear about what they want to evaluate; however,

---

Box 11.1 Questions about the evaluation

- What do you want to evaluate?
- Why are you undertaking the evaluation?
- Who is funding the evaluation?
- How do you intend to evaluate?
- Who will interpret the findings?
- How will findings be verified?
- How will the findings be used?
- What are the outcomes of evaluation for you or your organization?
- Who will benefit from the evaluation process?

---

clarity and reflection are also required as to why you want to undertake an evaluation. In essence, are you clear about the motivation behind your actions? Reflection can be described as thinking through a course of action before proceeding. It also involves revisiting decisions and actions, considering the associated thoughts and feelings and identifying the implications and outcomes of your action (Payne 2002, p.124). Reflective practice is key to maintaining ethical focus and should be implemented throughout the duration of the evaluation.

There are several reasons why an agency might support staff in the evaluation of a service. It is important to note that those reasons may not always be to the benefit of the individual who receives the service in question. For example, evaluation of a specific service may be initiated to meet policy guidance in a particular area (see Chapter 4). This consideration of the nature of the support that you receive also extends to who is funding the project and why.

The exact methodology to be applied is also extremely significant. For example, how will you select participants? When working with people who have dementia it is often necessary to reach them through negotiation with medical practitioners, families and ethics committees. This can be even more complicated when the potential participant is from a hidden population such as a minority ethnic background (Bowes and Wilkinson 2002).

The need to approach an ethics committee can be a time-consuming but essential exercise. Depending on the size of your project or where it is located this may also involve gaining the approval of more than one ethics committee. This should be viewed as a positive opportunity to demonstrate the safeguards that you will be applying and not as an obstacle or test. Barnett (2000, p.45) confirms this view advising that preparing an ethical protocol facilitated further consideration of practical issues and potential problems in her own evaluation into a health service facility for people with dementia. My own personal experience was also a valuable lesson in thinking through every aspect of an evaluation. I carried out an evaluation of the effects of a support and education group for people with dementia on issues of social inclusion and decision-making. In order to gain approval for my project I had to approach three ethics committees including the educational facility, the medical ethics committee and that of the local social work department. Each committee had interests in different aspects of the research and the methods that would be employed.

The range of methods that can be used in an evaluation require careful consideration prior to selection. With reference to my own experience in this area I designed a methodology to consider the effects of attending a time-limited support and education group for individuals with an early diagnosis of dementia. There was a particular focus on the effects of the group on social inclusion. For the purpose of the study decision-making was identified as an indicator of inclusion. I was motivated to consider this, as a literature review in this area informed me that previous research about group work appeared to focus on issues of well-being (Duff and Peach 1994; Gourlay and Short 1997).

The research participants consisted of the people who attended the group and a comparison group. As there was an open referral policy the group participants were recruited from a variety of sources. The comparison group consisted of individuals with an early diagnosis of dementia who had not attended a support and education group but were keen to do so. This group of participants were recruited through a local memory clinic. I approached the evaluation participants one and five months respectively after the termination of the group. The aims of the study were to identify the factors that affect decision-making and care-planning in the opinion of people with dementia. It also explored the role of group work in this process and other initiatives to promote decision-making by removing the barriers as identified by individuals with dementia. I considered the accounts of people with dementia to be an important data source in this evaluation. In order to elicit this information I utilized individual case studies and face-to-face interviews. Other methods however include questionnaires, telephone interviews, focus groups, observational studies and specific dementia tools such as dementia care mapping (Kitwood and Bredin 1992; Wilkinson 2002). Each method has particular implications for both the participant and the co-ordinator of the evaluation that require to be considered before selection. The particular bias that can occur in the person undertaking the study also interpreting the findings is also an issue for consideration. Transparency about how the findings will be used, verified and who will benefit from the process is therefore pivotal.

Accountability to the participant

Perhaps the most challenging question is that of consent. How will you ensure that the person with dementia wants to be included in your project? The ambiguity in this area is often seen as the main barrier to inclusion in the evaluation process. Consent from the family is also crucial; however, it is important to note that the approval of a relative or other independent source is not a legal substitute for the consent of the participant (Medical Research Council 1991). Alzheimer Scotland (2000) state that the two important principles of inclusion in research and evaluation are, first, whatever the degree of dementia, 'the person with dementia should be made aware, as far as possible, of what will be involved'. Second, if the person with dementia 'is not willing to participate then he or she should not be recruited to the research project (even if it is a relative's wish that the person takes part)'. Bartlett and Martin (2002, p.53) agree, advising that: 'Consent is a process of communication, of information and understanding, and effective family member (or surrogate) participation and co-operation.'

The components of consent have been identified by the Medical Research Council (1991) as:

- the provision of information

- the capacity to understand it

- the voluntary nature of agreed participation.

So how do you ascertain this? Box 11.2 outlines the essential elements of ethical practice in this area through demonstrated accountability to the participant.

Box 11.2 Essential elements in demonstrating accountability to the participant

- Information about the evaluation (see Box 11.1)
- A consent process
- Availability of independent advice and information
- Opt-out agreements
- Privacy/confidentiality safeguards
- Identified benefits to the person through participation
- No detriment to the person through inclusion or opt-out
- Feedback arrangements
- A complaints process

The provision of information is the first stage and can be achieved by spending time with potential participants and their families prior to the evaluation commencing. Information about the evaluation should be provided in a variety of formats for discussion and reference. Information should be provided in a format that can be interpreted by that particular participant. For example information can be broken down in small easy-to-read sections with clear headings and provided to the individual over an appropriate time frame. Information can also be provided in audio formats for individuals with dementia who are experiencing difficulty with reading or retaining the memory of written content. It is important to ensure that there is an available contact point for clarification or further discussion of the evaluation. In doing this the potential participant and their family or representative can obtain further information about the evaluation.

It is also useful to advise local and regional interest or advocacy groups such as Alzheimer Scotland about your evaluation. These groups can assist at many levels of the evaluation process. For example special interest groups can assist in identifying evaluation participants, give an opinion on the structure of your chosen evaluation or help participants understand what the proposed evaluation is about. Access for participants to an independent advocate or information source should be facilitated for the duration of the evaluation.

In order to provide informed consent the individual must understand the effects and implications of agreed participation before arriving at a decision. Given that each individual's pathway through the condition is different the ability to consent has to be considered in each instance. Competence has to be understood within specific contexts, choices and decisions (Goldsmith 1999; Kane 1998). Braye and Preston-Shoot advise that decision-making therefore has to be 'minutely dissected to maximise autonomy in those areas where competency can be established rather than operating on a blanket disqualification' (1993, p.127).

Consideration is therefore required of the person's ability to identify issues, form opinions and reach decisions in the subject area particular to the evaluation. The ability to retain the memory of views and to communicate these views are also important areas for consideration. Given the progressive nature of dementia, Reid, Ryan and Enderby (2001, p.382) advocate raising the issue of consent on each interaction with participants, referring to process consent (Usher and Arthur 1998). This approach revisits the issue of capacity to consent and agreement to participate throughout the evaluation and provides an important ethical safeguard. In all cases a written or verbal consent should be recorded in the presence of a relative or advocate.

Where a person does not have capacity to consent there is a strict legislative framework that must be applied. In Scotland this is provided by the Adults with Incapacity (Scotland) Act (2000) (Scottish Executive 2000). Part V of this Act advises that the permission of a recognized proxy such as a Welfare Power of Attorney or a Welfare Guardian can be given; however, engagement with the individual remains essential. Research on adults incapable of consenting is authorized under the Act provided that:

- it will further knowledge
- it is of benefit to the adult or others in a similar condition
- it entails little or no risk or discomfort
- the adult is not objecting
- consent has been obtained from a person with relevant powers
- the research has been approved by an appropriate ethics committee.

When undertaking any evaluation the relationship between the evaluator and the participant should be one of mutual trust (Bartlett and Martin 2002, p.48). Box 11.2 outlined the essential components of demonstrating accountability to participants in order to establish trust. It is important to ensure that potential participants and their families are aware that the decision to proceed with the project will not affect the service that they currently receive. For example if you are undertaking an evaluation of a day centre, can the participant offer a negative view without this adversely affecting the quality of the care provided in the future? Participants must also be offered the right to opt out of the evaluation at any time, again without detriment to the service that they currently receive. Transparency of process that can be discussed with an independent source is also a good way for the participant to consider if the evaluation is right for them. It is also essential to clarify the exact role and responsibility of the person undertaking the evaluation. For example, if a participant discloses a need that is not relevant to the evaluation what will you do with this information?

It is also essential that there is a transparent complaints process that the participant can access at any time. For example, in my own evaluation project information was given to each participant at the start of the process regarding the framework of accountability. If the participant or their family had any complaint or concern an independent approach could be made to either the educational facility that I was attached to or to the independent advocacy project. This was agreed with the advocacy project as part of my ethical committee submission and is a good example of the need to work in partnership with interest groups in order to maintain accountability to the participant. This is even more important when the evaluation is undertaken by the provider of the service in question as role ambiguity can be an issue for the evaluator as well as the participant. Creativity is often required on the part of the evaluator and/or employer in order to achieve transparency.

Ethics, participation and dementia

Box 11.3 refers to specific issues that must be addressed when undertaking evaluations involving people with dementia. The evaluation participants will have varying degrees of memory impairment. It is therefore important to plan your engagement to accommodate this. Given the possibility of memory loss, impaired judgement or insight (Jacques and Jackson 2000) can a person with dementia provide factual information? There will be occasions where participants will be unable to recall sources of information or details about their care or service received. Moyes (2001, p.41) advises that researchers should move from viewing this issue as one of 'them and us', preferring a perspective of the researcher as: 'Knowledgeable and sympathetic but lacking real insight [into the experience of having dementia].'

Box 11.3 Specific issues to be addressed in evaluations involving people with dementia

- Individual frameworks for information sharing
- Process consent (Usher and Arthur 1998)
- Legal safeguards
- Advocacy
- Engagement models
- Use of the word 'dementia'
- Hearing the voice of the participant (Goldsmith 1996)
- Allowing time

Individuals with dementia should be considered as: 'Skilled communicators who have real experience of the subject matter.' Many will be 'Keen, willing, vocal and [will have a] vested interest in seeing services improve' (Moyes 2001, p.41).

Given the likelihood that the person with dementia may experience some impairment of language, consideration is required to overcoming any barriers that this may present. Cox *et al.* (1998, p.9) remind us however that the reality is that the spoken and written word has a central role in expressing and understanding needs and views. Barnett (2000, p.47), referring to her own evaluation, describes a process of 'supporting the person through their own train of thought – even if I could not initially understand the relevance of what they said'.

When undertaking my own research I found discussion prompts to be useful in supporting the person with their train of thought. Others involved might require visual cues to assist with getting the message across. Behaviour is also a form of expression and communication (Cox *et al.* 1998). Time, expertise and knowledge of the person are required in understanding the informal cues exhibited by the person. Killick (1994) refers to this as creative listening. This part of the process can be time-consuming but essential if you are committed to inclusive practice. Participants may discuss experiences and emotions throughout the interaction as well as providing opinions. McKillop (2002, p.109), speaking as a person with dementia, describes his own participation in research as 'resurrecting bitter memories'. Building in time to deal with the potential for upset at emotional disclosures is essential. An awareness of how to ask questions in a way that is meaningful to participants is also required (Patton 1990). The use of language appropriate to demography and background is therefore pivotal.

The presence of a relative or advocate at interviews should be offered as the norm and arranged where this is the participant's choice. Discussions should always be held with the utmost sensitivity. If the evaluation requires specific discussion about the issue of dementia then this should be checked prior to recruiting each individual. Participants should be selected with a view to their willingness to discuss the issues related to the evaluation. However, it should also be agreed that interviews will be stopped if any upset is caused at discussion topics no matter what the timetable for the evaluation is. Participants should be aware that they are under no obligation to discuss topics raised and that any interview or interaction can be terminated at their request. The confidential nature of all information should also be explicit.

The venue for the evaluation interaction also needs to be considered. For example, an evaluation for a specific service may need to be undertaken at a specific venue for observational or contextual purposes. Wherever possible the interaction should take place at the venue that the individual prefers. Each interaction should be scheduled at the participant's convenience. This allows the participant to assert control over where and when the interaction will take place.

Written accounts are available about the effect of tiredness and optimum times for improved cognition when working with people with dementia (Davis 1989; Robinson 2002; Yale 1995). Robinson (2002, p.104) describes fluctuating episodes of confusion and advises: 'All I want to do is sleep and I'm afraid that when this happens everything just grinds to a halt for me.' Others refer to changing sleep patterns as the disease progresses (Davis 1989). Yale (1995, p.95) discusses the differences as to what works for each individual. In her experience of groupwork she found that some people tired in the afternoon and that some group participants appeared more confused later in the day. As a result differing appointment times will be required for participants in order to facilitate optimum participation. Appointments later in the day may also be anxiety-provoking. It is therefore essential to understand the person involved including personality traits and lifestyle preferences. This is invaluable in assisting the communication process (Murphy 1994) and creating a basis for trust. The duration of the interaction also needs consideration and should be agreed with the participant, their carer and advocate prior to beginning. It is also essential to build in time to confirm your role at the start of each interaction and confirm that consent is still given. Carers and family can offer insight into how the participant has been since the evaluation began and whether they believe that the person is happy to continue.

It is important to be aware that participation in an evaluation can be extremely disruptive to the individual and their family. It can also be physically and emotionally exhausting. Participants and carers therefore require the flexibility to cancel appointments and re-schedule even at very short notice. Again drawing on the experience of people who know what participation involves, Robinson (2002, p.105) describes days when she felt unable to take part in anything despite a willingness to contribute. It can however also be extremely rewarding. McKillop (2002, p.113) discusses his experience of participating in a research process as offering the opportunity to shape the future, benefit others, meet other people and most importantly offer a reflective opportunity to others on the subject of dementia.

Planning for the end of the evaluation is also essential. Each participant must be aware if the evaluation relationship will only last until the end of a particular project. If we consider dementia within a systems theory (Bronfenbrenner 1979; Sherlock and Gardiner 1996) of mutual interaction between the individual, the family, the community and wider society then the evaluator's presence, no matter how temporary, will impact on that system. Accountability and trust are demonstrated through endings which respect the fact that you have been allowed into an individual or family's life for even a short period of time. You should therefore be prepared to refer participants on to further contact points if any need is created through your own interaction. Feedback regarding the results and impact of the evaluation to the participant and their family is essential in retaining accountability to the participant throughout the life of the evaluation. Participants should be aware of when the evaluation outcome will be known. Findings should be reported to the person in a format that can be interpreted by that individual. Robinson states that 'It would be very disheartening for us to spend our time taking part in interviews or providing written material only to find that we would no longer hear from those conducting the research' (2002, p.106).

Ethical practice relies on an integral use of reflection. This should not only be evident throughout the duration of the project but should continue after the evaluation has ended. A review of the process employed should be considered in order to identify areas of practice or method that can be improved on. In this way a strong ethical base can be established for future evaluation projects.

Conclusion

This chapter has focused on the challenges in addressing the ethical implications of evaluation in dementia care. We make ethical decisions and choices every day. Ethics is central to who we are, what we do and how our society functions. People who have dementia are also members of society and have the same human rights as everyone else but can often find themselves waiting on others to include them or bestow their rights upon them. In the first section of this chapter the ethical principles associated with evaluation were discussed. The depersonalization and social isolation that people with dementia experience mean that ethical practice in evaluation refers to both the need to include and the need to safeguard. The vulnerability associated with dementia does necessitate safeguards in order to avoid exploitation and inappropriate practice. These safeguards exist to guide practice and are not intended to be barriers to inclusion. Ethical practice is therefore time-consuming and complex but essential. Ethical practice begins at the planning stage of the evaluation and continues throughout the life of the evaluation. It is apparent in how you select participants, how you engage with people and how you feed back to participants after the evaluation has ended. Reflective practice is central to maintaining a clear ethical focus. Goldsmith (1999, p.93) suggests that the ethical ambiguity that arises in working with people with dementia is often used as justification for the slow progress in facilitating inclusive practice. The challenge for anyone undertaking an evaluation with a person who has dementia is engaging in a way that demonstrates respect, accountability and a genuine willingness to spend the time in hearing the views of the individual with dementia. This chapter has attempted to assist this process by highlighting suggested good practice in this area. This in turn should ensure that our reflection of ourselves and our society does not make uncomfortable viewing.

References

Adams, T. and Clarke, C. (eds) (1999) *Dementia Care: Developing Partnerships in Practice.* London: Bailliere Tindall.

Alzheimer Scotland (2000) *Action on Dementia: Volunteering for Research into Dementia. Information Sheet 3.* Edinburgh: Alzheimer Scotland.

Banks, S. (2001) *Ethics and Values in Social Work.* London: Macmillan Press.

Barnett, E. (2000) *Including the Person with Dementia in Designing and Delivering Care: I Need to be Me.* London: Jessica Kingsley Publishers.

Bartlett, H. and Martin, W. (2002) 'Ethical issues in dementia care research.' In H. Wilkinson (ed.) *The Perspectives of People with Dementia: Research Methods and Motivations.* London: Jessica Kingsley Publishers.

Bowes, A. and Wilkinson, H. (2002) 'South Asian people with dementia: research issues.' In H. Wilkinson (ed.) *The Perspectives of People with Dementia: Research Methods and Motivations.* London: Jessica Kingsley Publishers.

Braye, S. and Preston-Shoot, M. (1993) 'Empowerment, partnership and mental health.' *Journal of Social Work Practice 7,* 2, 115–128.

Bronfenbrenner, U. (1979) *The Ecology of Human Development.* Cambridge, MA: Harvard University Press.

Cox, S., Anderson, I., Dick, S. and Elgar, J. (1998) *The Person, the Community and Dementia: Developing a Value Framework.* Stirling: Dementia Services Development Centre.

Davis, R. (1989) *My Journey into Alzheimer's Disease.* Amersham: Scripture Press.

Downie, R. and Telfer, E. (1980) *Caring and Curing: A Philosophy of Medicine and Social Work.* London: Methuen.

Duff, G. and Peach, E. (1994) *Mutual Support Groups: A Response to the Early and Often Forgotten Stages of Dementia.* Stirling: Dementia Services Development Centre.

Fontana, A. and Smith, R.W. (1989) 'Alzheimer disease victims: the "unbecoming" of self and the normalisation of competence.' *Sociological Perspectives 32,* 35–46.

Friel McGowan, D. (1993) *Living in the Labyrinth: A Personal Journey Through the Maze of Alzheimer's.* San Francisco: Elder Books.

Goldsmith, M. (1996) *Hearing the Voice of People with Dementia.* London: Jessica Kingsley Publishers.

Goldsmith, M. (1999) 'Ethical dilemmas.' In T. Adams and C.L. Clarke (eds) *Dementia Care: Developing Partnerships in Practice.* London: Bailliere Tindall.

Gourlay, G. and Short, S. (1997) *Evaluation of Self Support Group for People with Dementia (October – November, 1996).* Falkirk: Joint Dementia Initiative.

Harding, N. and Palfrey, C. (1997) *The Social Construction of Dementia: Confused Professionals?* London: Jessica Kingsley Publishers.

Hill, T.M. (1999) 'Western medicine and dementia: a deconstruction.' In T. Adams and C.L. Clarke (eds) *Dementia Care: Developing Partnerships in Practice.* London: Bailliere Tindall.

Jacques, A. and Jackson, G. (2000) *Understanding Dementia* (Third edition). Edinburgh: Churchill Livingstone.

Kane, M.N. (1998) 'Consent and competency in elders with Alzheimer's disease.' *American Journal of Alzheimer's Disease,* July/August, 179–188.

Killick, J. (1994) *Please Give Me Back My Personality.* Stirling: Dementia Services Development Centre.

King's Fund Centre (1986) *Living Well into Old Age: Applying Principles of Good Practice to Services for People with Dementia.* London: King's Fund Publishing Office.

Kitwood, T. (1996) 'The concept of personhood and its implications for the care of those who have dementia.' In G.M.M. Jones and B.M.L. Miesen (eds) *Care-giving in Dementia. Volume Two.* London: Routledge.

Kitwood, T. (1997) *Dementia Re-considered.* Buckingham: Open University Press.

Kitwood, T. and Bredin, K. (1992) 'A new approach to the evaluation of dementia care.' *Journal of Advances in Health and Nursing Care 1,* 5, 41–60.

McKillop, J. (2002) 'Did research alter anything?' In H. Wilkinson (ed.) *The Perspectives of People with Dementia: Research Methods and Motivations.* London: Jessica Kingsley Publishers.

Mark, R. (1996) *Research Made Simple: A Handbook for Social Workers.* London: Sage.

Martin, R.J. and Post, S.G. (1992) 'Human dignity, dementia and the moral basis of care-giving.' In R.H. Binstock, S.G. Post and P.J. Whitehouse (eds) *Dementia and Aging: Ethics, Values and Policy Choices.* Baltimore: Johns Hopkins University Press.

Medical Research Council (MRC) (1991) *The Ethical Conduct of Research on the Mentally Incapacitated.* London: MRC.

Moyes, M. (2001) 'The voice of the user group.' In C. Murphy, J. Killick and K. Allan (eds) *Hearing the User's Voice: Encouraging People with Dementia to Reflect on their Experiences of Services.* Stirling: Dementia Services Development Centre.

Murphy, C. (1994) *It Started with a Seashell: Life Story Work and People with Dementia.* Stirling: Dementia Services Development Centre.

Osborne, T. (1998) 'Constructionism, authority and the ethical life.' In I. Velody and R. Williams (eds) *The Politics of Constructionism.* London: Sage.

Patton, M.Q. (1990) *Qualitative Evaluation and Research Methods* (Second edition). Newbury Park, CA: Sage.

Payne, M. (2002) 'Social work theories and reflective practice.' In R. Adams, L. Dominelli and M. Payne (eds) *Social Work Theories, Themes, Issues and Critical Debates* (Second edition). Basingstoke: Palgrave.

Pratt, R. (2002) 'Nobody's ever asked how I felt.' In H. Wilkinson (ed.) *The Perspectives of People with Dementia: Research Methods and Motivations.* London: Jessica Kingsley Publishers.

Reid, D., Ryan, T. and Enderby, P. (2001) 'What does it mean to listen to people with dementia?' *Disability and Society 16,* 3, 377–392.

Robinson, E. (2002) 'Should people with Alzheimer's Disease take part in research?' In H. Wilkinson (ed.) *The Perspectives of People with Dementia: Research Methods and Motivations.* London: Jessica Kingsley Publishers.

Scottish Executive (2000) *Adults with Incapacity (Scotland) Act 2000.* Edinburgh: HMSO.

Sherlock, J. and Gardiner, I. (1996) 'Systematic family intervention.' In A. Chapman and M. Marshall (eds) *Dementia: New Skills for Social Workers. Case Studies for Practice 5.* London: Jessica Kingsley Publishers.

Usher, K.J. and Arthur, D. (1998) 'Process consent: a model for enhancing informed consent in mental health nursing.' *Journal of Advanced Nursing 27,* 692–697.

Wilkinson, H. (2002) 'Including people with dementia in research: methods and motivations.' In H. Wilkinson (ed.) *The Perspectives of People with Dementia: Research Methods and Motivations.* London: Jessica Kingsley Publishers.

Yale, R. (1995) *Developing Support Groups for Individuals with Early-Stage Alzheimer's Disease: Planning, Implementation and Evaluation.* Baltimore, MD: Health Promotions Press.

Chapter 12

User Involvement in Evaluations

Charlie Murphy

User involvement as applied to users of health and social welfare services generally was a radical concept at one time. Carr-Hill (1985) described it as 'the view from underneath' (p.373). Things have progressed from that in a western culture where the pre-eminence of the role of the consumer has made its way into the health and social welfare field. In particular the learning disabilities field has many lessons to teach those who work with people with dementia. It has generally preceded that of dementia in terms of innovative thinking and practice. The issue of user involvement, especially in research and evaluation, is no exception to this principle. Ritchie (1996) speaks of the involvement of people with learning disabilities in aspects of the research and evaluation process.

User involvement' as applied to evaluation in the learning disabilities field has encompassed asking users about services, having users involved as interviewers, and having users involved in the design phase of service evaluations (see March, Steingold and Justice 1997; Ritchie 1996; Stenfert Kroese, Gillott and Atkinson 1998; Walmsley and Johnson 2003, pp.95–108, 109–125; Whittaker, Gardner and Kershaw 1991). This extensive interpretation of 'involvement' does not apply yet where people with dementia are concerned. Indeed it is only recently that the idea of asking individuals with dementia about services that they (had) received began to be taken seriously. Cheston and Bender (2000) in their review of this area cite only a handful of published examples. Prior to this the views of individuals with dementia were traditionally 'heard' through the comments of relatives or professionals speaking on their behalf. The 1990s saw prominence given to observational approaches, and in particular Dementia Care Mapping (DCM) (Bradford Dementia Group 1997; Brooker 2001).

In this chapter I wish to cover three aspects of hearing users' views – practical and logistical considerations; ethical challenges; and finally, a discussion of how users' views fit into an evaluation context. The presentation will rely on a number of evaluations in which I have been involved in the period 1996 to 2004. These evaluations involved day care projects (Murphy 2004; Murphy, Glover and Davis 1996); a befriending scheme; a community dementia team; an advocacy project (Murphy 2001); an early stage support group (Murphy 2004); the use of reminiscence; and also the use of life storybooks (Murphy 2000b). As some of these evaluations were internal commissions there is no associated published work. Predominantly the methods adopted for hearing the views of people with dementia were interviews, most of which were semi-structured.

Practical and logistical considerations

There are seven personal 'guidelines', which I have developed to assist me in hearing the views of individuals with dementia in service evaluations. Some of these represent good practice generally for interviewing situations. These guidelines are:

1. Establish a relationship with the person.

2. View the interaction more as a conversation than as an interview.

3. Be prepared to abandon the interview if necessary.

4. Prioritize the relationship-building over the asking of questions.

5. Maximize the 'immediacy' of what is being evaluated.

6. Maximize the communicative environment for the person with dementia.

7. Obtain as much of the factual information as possible in advance.

Establish a relationship with the person

As an external evaluator I have found it very important to establish a relationship with the individuals with dementia who may be interviewed. This is similar to the approach advocated by Tom Kitwood to enable staff to adopt person-centred care practice in their work (Kitwood 1997). In day care *establishing a relationship* may involve visiting the service in advance on one or two occasions, and taking part in the programme of activities. For both the reminiscence evaluation and the evaluation of the early stage support group this preliminary work to establish relationships involved sitting in on two sessions. In some evaluation circumstances it will be easier to do this than in others; for example, it was more difficult in the evaluation of one-to-one services such as advocacy (Murphy 2001) and befriending (Murphy 1997). There are potential time and cost implications in this approach which may be over and above those incurred in evaluating services for people who do not have dementia. We will return to this later.

View the interaction more as a conversation than as an interview

For individuals with dementia I believe that it is very important to view the process as more akin to a conversation rather than an interview (see also Patton 2002). Many people with dementia can feel under pressure when asked direct questions in a formal fashion. The process could then seem closer to a test. The evaluation interviews are designed to hear the *opinions* of the person with dementia, and this is what is stressed to the interviewee. Consequently the interviews are not seen as focusing on the recall of facts. These opinion questions can thus be woven into a format which is more discursive than interrogative. Another approach which I use to relax the person with dementia and decrease their anxiety is to reiterate that they are in fact helping me through their participation.

Be prepared to abandon the interview if necessary and prioritize the relationship-building over the asking of questions

It may be that in some circumstances the person with dementia is too agitated (or becomes too agitated) for the interview to proceed. This has only occurred to me once in over 50 interviews. The incident took place during an earlier evaluation – of a befriending service. The interview took place in the person's own home. Unfortunately the person with dementia barely sat down during the first 15 minutes that I was there. Many precautions had been taken. These included writing in advance to the person on distinctive coloured paper to request their participation; having someone familiar to the person explain the letter and what was involved in taking part in the evaluation; making a reminder phone call shortly before my visit; and dressing informally and casually for the interview. However, this woman was simply not comfortable with having visitors to her house and was anxious despite these precautions. Consequently the interaction that took place was closer to a life story or reminiscence conversation. Information on what the interviewee did during the war was forthcoming, for example. No pressure was exerted to take part in an interview process. This example also illustrates the fourth guideline about prioritizing relationship-building over asking questions.

Maximize the 'immediacy' of what is being evaluated

The difficulties which individuals with dementia may have with short-term memory and orientation are well documented. The fifth guideline therefore concerns 'immediacy' – a concept which I apply to both time and place. For example, in the evaluation of many of the day care projects, the interviews/discussions with members have taken place in a quiet room at the familiar day care venue, during the person's usual day at the day centre. This combination of both physical and temporal immediacy is not always possible. In the early stage support group evaluation interviews took place in a room next to where the group had met, but the interviews took place a week or two after the last meeting of the group. In the reminiscence project most interviews took place at the venue for the reminiscence sessions, shortly after a session had finished. One interview for the reminiscence project evaluation did take place while seated at the back of the project minibus, in hushed tones, as the person in question returned home at the end of the day. It was felt that this opportunism was important in order to maintain the immediacy of time for the individual. In the interviews for the befriending service a variety of approaches were adopted (Murphy 1997). On some occasions I took part in the befriending visit or outing and then interviewed the service user following that. In one instance the befriender left the service user and myself alone during the outing to have our discussion.

Immediacy was much more difficult to achieve with the evaluation of the advocacy project (Murphy 2001) and with the community dementia team evaluation (Murphy and Cox 2000). Indeed the advocacy evaluation presented numerous challenges and was perhaps the least successful of all in incorporating the views of people with dementia. A major difficulty arose in getting across the idea of advocacy in the first place. Photographs of the advocate were used in some instances to prompt the person with dementia, although this was not always successful. In many cases the advocacy intervention itself was over so immediacy was not possible.

Maximize the communicative environment for the person with dementia

The penultimate guideline refers to the need to maintain good communication practice with individuals with dementia in the evaluation interview situation. One should speak fairly slowly and convey small amounts of information at a time, for example. Also a more domestic and relaxing environment will help the person to relax, to be themselves and to communicate better. As an example, in the evaluation of the early stage support group the interview room was made to resemble a sitting room. Table lamps, coffee tables and a tray of tea and biscuits were some key ingredients in this process.

Another aspect of the environment is the social environment and the people involved in carrying out the interviews. A central consideration is whether to have an internal or external evaluator. The advantages of the former are that it will help the person with dementia to feel more relaxed (and probably cost less to the organization concerned). What is lost is an element of objectivity. In one of the early evaluations in which I was involved we were very fortunate to be able to engage the services of a peripatetic arts worker who was independent of the project being evaluated but who had worked with the members previously. Predominantly however the model I have used has been that of external evaluator building up a relationship with those being interviewed. In the learning disabilities field it is recommended that those carrying out evaluation interviews satisfy three criteria. These are that the interviewers are: local, sensitive, and trained.

One successful strategy, which I have developed for making the most out of the (social) environment, is to interview people with dementia in pairs. This approach was used very effectively in the evaluation of the early stage support group (Murphy 2004). The option of being interviewed in pairs was put to the participants and most indicated a preference for this. One immediate benefit is the availability of peer support through having another person with dementia present. Those taking part can identify with each other when they cannot find the right word or when they forget what they were going to say. Thus the moment is less embarrassing or stigmatizing.

Deciding on the number of questions to ask or the number of issues to address are important considerations in the process of maintaining a good communicative environment. Allowing oneself time to pilot the interview schedule can be very helpful. This was the case with the interviews for the befriending evaluation. As a result of the pilot interview a schedule of 25 questions was reduced to five issues. Interestingly a longer schedule was used for the interviews in the evaluation of the early stage support group. This was because other factors supported this – relationships had been established over a longer time; the environment was very non-threatening; and the interviewees had peer support.

Obtain as much of the factual information as possible in advance

Finally it can help the interview process to have gathered some relevant factual information from other evaluation sources prior to the interviews. For example, in the befriending interviews, the volunteer befrienders had been interviewed prior to the service users. This meant that any indirect references to aspects of the befriending outing could be picked up as the background was already familiar to the interviewer. Also for the advocacy evaluation, the interviews with service users predominantly took place after those with other stakeholders to ensure that the interviewer had as much background information as possible.

Ethical considerations

The focus of this section is on ethical considerations when attempting to involve service users. These are:

- consent
- intrusion
- expectations
- tokenism
- interpretation
- confidentiality versus responsibility
- reciprocity
- implications of non-involvement.

For a fuller discussion of ethical issues involved in evaluating dementia care in general see Chapter 11.

Consent

Questions which need to be addressed under this heading include who asks for the consent, when to ask and how to ask. On some occasions it has been project staff who have explained the evaluation and asked for consent (for example, Murphy 1997; Murphy and Cox 2000); on others it has been the interviewer (Murphy 2000a; Murphy *et al.* 1996). The person with dementia should be provided with an information sheet written in accessible language using fairly large print. This information sheet or leaflet can explain what the evaluation involves; why it is taking place; and how it might benefit the individual and/or others with dementia. This leaflet should also discuss specific issues such as confidentiality and the right of the service user to withdraw from the process at any point. It can clarify that refusal to participate will not impact on the individual's receipt of services; and neither will any negative comments which are made about the service.

This is the process for getting initial consent – both verbally and in writing. However, evaluators and interviewers need to be alive to the spirit of consent and to whether consent is ongoing. Although consent has been given at one point in time, confirmation may be needed, at the start of the interview for example. Ongoing consent issues can be addressed with the help of non-verbal communication skills. Are there signs of agitation, lack of interest or disengagement from the person? These signs can be used to indicate whether an interview should start or not; but also whether it should continue. In one instance, from my own experience, a woman being interviewed about day care kept looking out the window of the room to a man outside watching cars in the car park. When I commented on the man, the service user replied 'He's nosey…just like you!', which was a fairly direct indication that the interview had become too intrusive and/or gone on for too long.

Intrusion

A colleague once stated that 'it is not that people with dementia come into our lives, but we enter into their lives'. Thus it is not that they will necessarily have a sound grasp of the different professional boundaries involved in health and social care, for example, and the role that we play within that. Rather we, as evaluators in this instance, interrupt the daily routine of the person with dementia and their carers, perhaps representing just another 'intruder' from a long list of those providing various services. There is a risk of upsetting the routines that people might have. This is one reason that the relationship-building which was referred to previously can be so important. It may be hard for evaluators to acknowledge that sometimes evaluations have been carried out simply for their own sake; that is, without any practical consequences for the interviewee or people with dementia generally. The problems of intrusion will not have been addressed in such instances. I feel it is a vitally important ethical consideration to have minimized disruption and intrusion and to have balanced any disruption or intrusion with a high degree of applicability and relevance for the piece of evaluation work.

Sometimes hands-on staff can act as gatekeepers to the individuals with dementia. Such actions may be driven by a desire to protect the person with dementia from unnecessary intrusion, or perhaps by a concern that the evaluator is not sufficiently skilled in working with people with dementia. On the other hand the gatekeeping may be motivated by a belief that the person with dementia cannot communicate their feelings about the service they receive (Goldsmith 1996). In the latter circumstance the workers' responses may indirectly contribute to the evaluation findings – for example, the need for training for such staff in person-centred approaches.

A final scenario to consider under the heading of intrusion is when a service is clearly in need of reform and change, probably before the evaluation has started. There might be a case for excluding people with dementia (not intruding) at this stage, if there is going to be a further evaluation and their involvement at this point might not add anything to what we know already of an under-performing service.

Expectations

There may be an unintentional consequence of establishing relationships with individuals with dementia for the purposes of an evaluation; and of recognizing that we enter their lives, rather than the reverse. It could be that the person with dementia does not appreciate that the relationship is time-limited, or it may be that the evaluator/interviewer develops a friendship which he or she may find hard to terminate. Consequently there may be expectations of an ongoing relationship. This issue is faced by hands-on workers frequently. It emphasizes the importance of clarity of communication by the evaluator from the beginning. It also points up the need to reinforce the message about the nature of the evaluation intervention on a regular basis. In one instance – during the life storybook evaluation (Murphy 2000b) – I did find myself revisiting an evaluation site for a social/personal visit to a participant.

Tokenism

Tokenism can work in two ways. It can involve asking individuals with dementia for their opinions but then not responding to any negative comments and not acting on criticisms. On the other hand it might mean interviewing some service users simply in order to cherry-pick positive comments for an annual report for example. How do we avoid tokenism? One step is to ensure that there is a willingness to act and/or change from both service managers and staff. This should be transparent from the beginning of an evaluation. It is important that such points are clarified at the early stages of the evaluation.

Interpretation

The responses by service users in interviews are not always clear-cut and unambiguous. In Keegan (1998) a nurse discovered that the apparently confused conversations which she was having with a patient with dementia made sense when the patient's responses were placed alongside the nurse's comments from a few minutes previously. In other words they were time delayed. Also it has been established that sometimes people with dementia may use words in a metaphorical fashion (see Killick 1994). In one of the early evaluations in which I was involved a day centre member talked about the benefits of doing exercises thus – 'it takes the wrinkles out of your bones'. This was not only poetic, but also witty.

One consequence of the above is that the interviewer may be adding his or her interpretation to the responses received. In one instance I interviewed a woman who talked about *learning the system* when asked if there was any advice that she would give to the workers at the day centre – 'They have to be good at learning the system, really good when they are talking.' This woman had used this turn of phrase previously in the interview. In the previous context it appeared to be a reference to how people communicated or got on together, and so that interpretation was applied when the phrase was used again.

Likewise a man interviewed for the befriending project (Murphy 1997) – when asked if he felt that he had benefited – replied that 'It gets me out of the house; to get me to be the same...' This last expression left room for interpretation – was the person with dementia meaning the same as he had been, or the same as everyone else, or the same as the befriender? From other replies which this person had given the interpretation 'gets me to be the same (as I have been)' makes most sense. Good practice in interpretation is to explain ambiguities and how they were resolved.

Confidentiality versus responsibility

There may be issues raised during evaluation interviews which the person would like to have addressed sooner rather than later. As mentioned earlier in this chapter it is we who enter the lives of individuals with dementia and not they who enter our lives. For example, a day centre member may not realize that their interview is part of a larger information-gathering process which will also include analysis and writing up a report. They might feel that a comment they have made, about lunch, for example, will be acted on immediately because it has been heard by someone official (in this case the evaluator). This reinforces the need for clarity of communication by the interviewer and between the interviewer and respondent. It highlights the need for the interviewer to be checking back with the person with dementia about their understanding of what will happen with their comments. And it may be in some instances that comments need to be acted upon sooner rather than later, especially if more serious allegations have been made. In such cases the evaluator/interviewer must be prepared to step outside their formal role. Indeed for some situations the evaluator may have to make the decision themselves when it is unclear whether the person wishes immediate action.

Reciprocity

Interviewing people with dementia for a service evaluation can be viewed as intruding into their lives and taking their opinions in order to add to the quality of the evaluation report. What will the person themselves get back, and if not an individual benefit then what will future service users gain? Ideally these questions will be addressed in any information leaflet produced for the evaluation. However, the questions should serve as further motivation for the evaluator to look at what is being offered to the person with dementia in return for their participation. Have those conducting the evaluation gained a commitment to change from staff; have they built in enough time to allow the person to express their views as best they can; and have they built in enough time to analyse and interpret what has been said as sensitively and accurately as possible? The readers may wish to compare comments by Patton on participation and collaboration in evaluation (2002, pp.182–185).

Another consideration, in terms of reciprocity, is whether evaluation findings can be made available to people with dementia who have taken part, if this is appropriate. The same guidelines on accessibility of language would apply as when the information sheet was discussed under 'consent' earlier.

Implications of non-involvement

The previous sections looked at ethical challenges in involving service users. Although there are many, and some challenges do demand sophisticated responses from evaluators, it is important to consider what we are saying if we choose not to include the views of people with dementia in an evaluation. Would we exclude any other group of service users in a similar situation, and if not then what justification is there in this instance? Ultimately excluding people with dementia from an evaluation may say more about the project and about the evaluation itself than any glossy report.

Users' views in an evaluation context

This chapter concludes with a discussion on the role of service users' views in an overall evaluation context, having previously discussed practical suggestions of how to gather such views and the ethical issues to take on board in this process. The positive contributions which listening to service users make to an evaluation include the following:

- We obtain the user's construction of what is successful rather than an external one.

- We can expect that the service user does not bring any professional bias to their opinion.

- We hear the views of the ultimate recipient (in this case the service user) which is invaluable in a service evaluation.

In some of the evaluations which I have undertaken the users' responses have highlighted different outcomes for people with dementia than service providers might have intended; there have been different constructions of 'success'. Barbara Lee speaks powerfully of 'insider' and 'outsider' perspectives in her contribution to Patton's book (Patton 2002, pp.333–338). Øvretveit also refers to the differing perspectives of different interest groups (1998, pp.49–52). From my own experience in day care programmes, service providers often focus on having a range of activities available to offer stimulation. Service users, however, often stress the social aspect of attending day care rather than specific activities (Murphy *et al.* 1996). This finding might encourage providers to put the 'process' before the 'task', since members, generally speaking, appeared more interested in simply 'being' and socializing with other people than the specific activity around which they were socializing.

These positive contributions to the whole evaluation do not come without their cost. Some of the additional costs incurred in asking people with dementia about the services that they receive have already been referred to. First, there are the additional resources involved in this process due to allocating time for relationship-building and focusing more on the conversational than the interrogative during the time spent with service users. Other costs might be incurred through extra services being deemed necessary following this evaluation exercise.

While allowing for the benefits of involving service users in evaluation there are a number of qualifications to be made when incorporating these views into an evaluation. The first factor to be aware of is that the respondent's dependency on the service that is being evaluated may impact on how critical he or she can be – this is irrespective of whether the person has dementia or not. In my experience of evaluations users are rarely critical, even when there are clear flaws in how the service is delivered. Some appear grateful for any service, for example they are pleased that a bus picks them up and returns them home from day care, even though this day care experience itself may be lacking in stimulation and may not be person-centred.

A second factor may be loyalty to a particular worker within a service which prevents criticism of the service itself. Also a small number of interviewees have pointed out that as a service user they do not have anything with which to compare the service that they are receiving, for example they will not have attended a number of support groups, or been to different day centres. Finally evaluators should be aware that service users will often find it easier to comment on the process of receiving a service rather than the outcome of it.

For all of the above reasons evaluations should try not to rely exclusively on the views of service recipients without some other measures to supplement that data. The most common of these are either observational or third party approaches, such as asking a third party about the impact of the service on the individual with dementia. A third party might include a family carer or a referring professional. In those evaluations where observational methods have been used they have often highlighted additional areas for improvement not identified by the respondents themselves. Also an observational approach might allow us to capture the perspective of non-respondents, service users who were not interviewed. In an early evaluation (Murphy *et al.* 1996), three day centre members declined to be interviewed, but did take part in a DCM exercise. Although the interviews were predominantly positive the DCM showed that these three non-respondents (plus the woman who commented unfavourably in the interviews) had lower well/ill-being scores (a coding frame indicating if a person is in a state of well-being or ill-being). In this observation the non-respondents were quieter, and tended to be excluded by volunteers at the day centre, many of whom may have struggled with how to communicate with them. All of which led to these members having a poorer experience. Observation methods were necessary to supplement the service users' views in this instance.

The use of third party approaches, for example asking for the opinions of referrers and/or relatives, may also plug some gaps in information from the service user interviews. In my experience these gaps have included outcomes which the individual with dementia has not remembered to say:

for example, rediscovering an old pastime with a befriender; being more alert on returning home from day care; or being more settled after day care.

Conclusion

This chapter has presented approaches from my experience which may help the reader to ensure that service users' views are incorporated into an evaluation in the best way possible. I have also introduced some of the ethical considerations which need to be reflected upon throughout such a process, especially the balance between intrusion and the need for/use of the evaluation itself. Finally the role which user views may play in an evaluation context has been examined for both its positive and negative facets.

References

Bradford Dementia Group (1997) *Evaluating Dementia Care: The DCM Method* (Seventh edition). Bradford: University of Bradford. (Available only as part of basic DCM course.)

Brooker, D. (2001) 'Enriching lives: evaluation of the ExtraCare activity challenge.' *Journal of Dementia Care 9*, 3, 33–37.

Carr-Hill, R.A. (1985) 'The evaluation of health care.' *Social Science and Medicine 21*, 4, 367–375.

Cheston, R. and Bender, M. (2000) 'Involving people who have dementia in the evaluation of services: a review.' *Journal of Mental Health 9*, 5, 471–479.

Goldsmith, M. (1996) *Hearing the Voice of People with Dementia.* London: Jessica Kingsley Publishers.

Keegan, C. (1998) *Talking with Jean.* Stirling: Dementia Services Development Centre.

Killick, J. (1994) 'There's so much to hear when you stop and listen to individual voices.' *Journal of Dementia Care 2*, 5, 16–17.

Kitwood, T. (1997) *Dementia Reconsidered: The Person Comes First.* Buckingham: Open University Press.

March, J., Steingold, B. and Justice, S. (1997) 'Follow the yellow brick road! People with learning difficulties as co-researchers.' *British Journal of Learning Disabilities 25*, 77–80.

Murphy, C.J. (1997) *An Evaluation of the Town Break Befriending Service.* Stirling: DSDC.

Murphy, C.J. (2000a) *An Evaluation of the Edinburgh Saturday Break.* Stirling: DSDC.

Murphy, C. (2000b) *'Crackin' Lives': An Evaluation of a Life Story Book Project to Assist Patients from a Long-stay Psychiatric Hospital in their Move to Community Care Situations.* Stirling: DSDC.

Murphy, C. (2001) *Evaluation of the Beth Johnson Foundation: Advocacy and Dementia Project 1998–2001.* Stirling: DSDC.

Murphy, C. (2004) *An Evaluation of an Early Stage Support Group for People with Dementia.* Stirling: DSDC.

Murphy, C. and Cox, S. (2000) *An Evaluation of Ross-shire Community Dementia Team.* (Unpublished.)

Murphy, C., Glover, M. and Davis, K. (1996) *An Evaluation of Stirling Town Break.* Stirling: DSDC.

Øvretveit, J. (1998) *Evaluating Health Interventions.* Buckingham: Open University Press.

Patton, M.Q. (2002) *Qualitative Research and Evaluation Methods.* Thousand Oaks: Sage.

Ritchie, P. (1996) 'Involving service users.' In R. McConkey (ed.) *Innovations in Evaluating Services for People with Intellectual Disabilities.* Chorley: Lisieux Hall Publications. pp.91–102.

Stenfert Kroese, B., Gillott, A. and Atkinson, V. (1998) 'Consumers with intellectual disabilities as service evaluators.' *Journal of Applied Research in Intellectual Disabilities 11,* 116–128.

Walmsley, J. and Johnson, K. (2003) *Inclusive Research with People with Learning Disabilities: Past, Present and Futures.* London: Jessica Kingsley Publishers.

Whittaker, A., Gardner, S. and Kershaw, J. (1991) *Service Evaluation by People with Learning Difficulties.* London: King's Fund Centre.

Chapter 13

Evaluation of Dementia Care in Resource-Scarce Settings

Jurate Macijauskiene

This chapter considers the challenges inherent in evaluating dementia care in resource-scarce settings using Lithuania, a new member of the European Union (EU), as an example. It begins by outlining care provision in Lithuania and thus providing a context in which resource-scarce evaluations take place. The chapter then proceeds using examples from the Lithuanian experience to discuss a number of key issues. These include: difficulties in ascertaining the size of an ageing population and identifying and diagnosing those who may have dementia, new and immature policy directives, economic restraints, lack of facilities and shortage of training.

With increasing numbers of older people, specific age-related conditions have become important around the globe. Every chronic disease and disability challenges health and social care systems, demanding economic provision and human resources. The financial consequences of population ageing are affecting health care systems in many countries, and many systems are in a state of more or less constant reorganization and restructuring (de Exter *et al.* 2004; Knapp 1995). Dementia can be distinguished from other age-related conditions by a number of factors, including its progressive nature and the importance of non-pharmacological measures and caregiving during the course of the disease.

Services for people with dementia vary greatly across different countries, not only due to different levels of economic development but also because of different national policies, infrastructures, and cultural distinctions. More developed countries have more comprehensive dementia care, although lack of continuity of care and adequate resources are identified as one of the major problems even among the countries of the European Union (Warner *et al.* 2002). However, longer established European Union members have long and interesting experience in establishing service provision for people with dementia and their caregivers. Those regions where dementia services are in the process of being developed can derive benefit from the constant development of health care and social service systems and increasing access to comprehensive diagnosing and effective treatment in more prosperous countries, as well as potentially learning from successful and efficient service models in those countries.

In the context of care for people with dementia all countries can be grouped according to their welfare systems and services for this group into one of three categories: (1) more developed countries with developed services; (2) more developed countries with developing services; (3) less developed countries with developing services. Lithuania is an example of a more developed country with developing services for people with dementia. After becoming a member of the EU in 2004, one of Lithuania's goals is to meet the recommended requirements for the care of their people. The transitional period in Lithuania, which started with the state regaining independence from the former Soviet Union in 1990, has markedly influenced demographic process, living conditions, health care system, and social provision. Table 13.1 presents the main socio-economic data for Lithuania compared to the average of 25 EU countries.

Table 13.1 indicates that the percentage of older people and old-age dependency ratios in Lithuania and in other EU countries when averaged are similar. Lithuania, like many European countries, is faced with the problem of an ageing population. Life expectancy in Lithuania as in many other new EU members is lower than that in longer established EU members for a number of reasons. Economic conditions are different. Based on World Bank 2004 criteria Lithuania is one of the higher middle-income group countries. To put this in a European context, Lithuania's per capita GDP has increased consistently; however, it is still only 50 per cent of the EU average. Additionally the percentage of GDP devoted to

Table 13.1 The main socio-economic characteristics of Lithuania

	Lithuania	EU25 average
Demographics		
Population	3.4 mln[1]	–
Percentage of older people (aged 65+ years)	15.1[1]	16.3[2]
Old-age dependency ratio	37.3[2]	38.8[2]
Life expectancy		
At birth (men, women)	66.3, 77.5[2]	74.8, 81.1[2]
At 65 (men, women)	13.3, 17.7[2]	16.0, 19.6[2]
Economics		
Gross domestic product (GDP) per capita (in 2003)[2]	50.1	100
Share of social protection expenditure of GDP, percentage (in 2001)[3]	15.2	27.3
Health expenditure as percentage of GDP[3]	4.3	6.6
Per capita total expenditure on health in international dollars (in 2002)	549[4]	2128[5]

EU25 – European Union including all 25 countries
1 Department of Statistics of the Government of the Republic of Lithuania, 2005
2 GDP per capita = GDP in 2004 in Purchasing Power Standards in relation to EU25 (EU25=100)
    average; source: EUROSTAT 2005
3 Source: EUROSTAT 2005
4 WHO Statistical Information System (WHOSIS 2002)
5 OECD Health Data 2004, First edition, WHO Regional Office for Europe

social expenditure in Lithuania is less than half the average for all EU countries.

The more developed, highly industrialized countries of Europe and North America are home to most of the world's oldest populations. That said, even in countries that, according to the ageing index, are young, the absolute numbers of older people in less developed countries are large and increasing. Currently 59 per cent of the world's older people live in less developed countries (Kinsella and Velkoff 2001). As a result of demographic ageing processes by 2020 the oldest sector of the population will have increased by 200 per cent in less developed countries compared with 68 per cent in the more developed world (WHO and WFN 2004). This puts considerable pressure on less developed countries' economies and public health provision. Countries with low-income economies are forced to confront the challenges in health and social care sectors and inequalities in allocating very scarce resources.

Dementia statistics

Dementia statistics have three major features. First, there are no population-based dementia studies on people over 65 in many countries, including Lithuania and 15 other EU countries (Berr, Wancata and Ritchie 2005). Based on the number of cases registered by the State Mental Health Centre of Lithuania, there has been a considerable increase in cases of dementia and Alzheimer's disease, probably due to improved access to services and better recognition (Puras *et al.* 2004; WHO 2005). According to Ona Davidoniene, Director of State Mental Health Centre, Lithuania, in 2004 there were 808 registered cases of Alzheimer's disease and 14,534 registered cases of vascular and other dementias (Personal communication 2005). Using figures from a Rotterdam study (Breteler, Ott and Hofman 1998; Ott *et al.* 1995), Macijauskiene and Engedal (2005) have roughly estimated the true prevalence of dementia in Lithuania to be around 31,000 cases with an annual incidence of around 6000 new cases. However, given that life expectancy, prevalence of disorders and living conditions are different in different countries, estimates based on calculations from the Rotterdam study are not reliable. Also, the proportions of various types of dementia in Lithuania may be different from those of other countries. Other epidemiological studies (Ott *et al.* 1995; Suh and Shah 2001) indicate that the majority of dementia in many countries is due to Alzheimer's disease whereas a comparatively small proportion of all dementia is attributed to Alzheimer's disease in Lithuania. It has been reported that vascular dementia is more prevalent than Alzheimer's disease in India (Jha and Patel 2004). Epidemiological studies might reveal the proportions of different types of dementias, with Lithuanian data differing from that for other countries (Fratiglioni *et al.* 1991; Ott *et al.* 1995; Suh and Shah

2001). Further, there are no data on the severity of dementia in Lithuania. Such data could be helpful in planning health and social care services, although the degree of dementia alone is not the best indicator of the need for institutional care (Alzheimer Scotland 2000).

In less developed countries, there is even more uncertainty over the prevalence of dementia, with few studies and varying estimates, although the evidence suggests that the prevalence and incidence of dementia is lower than in more developed countries (10/66 Dementia Research Group 2004; Alvarado-Esquil *et al.* 2004). There is a need for further epidemiological research on dementia, particularly in Latin America, Russia and Eastern Europe, the Middle East, and Africa (Ferri *et al.* 2005).

Health and social care provision

Health and social care provision and the provision of specialist dementia care vary greatly from country to country, with a spectrum that runs from almost exclusively family care in less developed countries to high institutionalization rates in more developed countries (Burns, O'Brien and Ames 2005). Within the EU, dementia care models are quite advanced in some countries but in the early stages of development in others (Warner *et al.* 2002).

Lithuania is in the process of organizing health and social services for older people, particularly for those with dementia. Specialists (neurologists, psychiatrists and, rarely, geriatricians) employed in the 'secondary' or 'tertiary' service sectors perform diagnoses and assessments of dementia following referrals from general practitioners or other specialists. When both the diagnosis and the cause of dementia are confirmed, specific treatment and risk prevention services become available. It is important to diagnose dementia earlier, since the newest and specific treatment strategies are available in Lithuania, although the costs of drug-based treatments are not fully met by the state. Further medical management of people with dementia is being conducted mainly by psychiatrists, neurologists, and few geriatricians. Primary mental health care is provided by a team of specialists (a psychiatrist, a mental health nurse, a social worker and a psychologist) in primary mental health centres with countrywide coverage. These centres ensure medical treatment, primary diagnosis of dementia, family consultations, the management of social and psychological problems and visits to homes when needed. Although health and social needs are being assessed, such assessments do not result in comprehensive care plans for people with dementia due to lack of services and institutions. In rural areas, people with dementia are mainly cared for by general practitioners and community nurses.

Institutional services

For the whole of Lithuania there are four psychogeriatric departments with a total of 115 beds dedicated to caring for older people with psychiatric disorders and people with dementia with exacerbated emotional and behavioural problems. If there is no access to specialized psychogeriatric care, people with dementia are admitted to acute psychiatric units. Nursing hospitals can provide short-term nursing care (maximum length of stay is four months). The number of beds in nursing hospitals has increased threefold between 1995 and 2001 but these hospitals lack dementia-specific units. Those who live alone and need permanent social and medical care are accommodated in state care institutions for older people or care institutions for mentally disabled adults, which cater for all age groups. As from 2005 there were 22 long-care institutions for mentally disabled adults in Lithuania with a total of 5309 residents (Department of Audit and Supervision of Social Establishments at the Ministry of Social Security and Labour 2005). People with dementia constituted 8.4 per cent of all residents in these institutions. In state care institutions for older people, people with dementia make up to 22.1 per cent of all residents (Department of Audit and Supervision of Social Establishments at the Ministry of Social Security and Labour 2005). The research literature suggests that many countries have higher proportions of people with dementia in nursing homes for older people than Lithuania, with percentages from 26.4 per cent to 74 per cent (Engedal and Haugen 1993; Melzer et al. 2004; O'Brien and Caro 2001). However, a recent study by Alvarado-Esquil et al. reported 16.1 per cent of residents with dementia in nursing homes in Mexico (Alvarado-Esquil et al. 2004). Summarizing, the numbers of people with dementia in Lithuania living in long-term care institutions amount to around 2 per cent of the estimated actual numbers of people with dementia. Thus, in Lithuania people with dementia are mainly being cared for at home and by their relatives. Very few long-term care institutions are designed for the needs of people with dementia.

Regardless of how many persons with different degrees of dementia there are in Lithuania, the numbers catered for by the respective institutions and services are too low. A relatively low percentage of older people in Lithuania receive permanent long-term care services compared to other European countries – 0.9 per cent in Lithuania compared to 6–10 per cent elsewhere in Europe (Government of Lithuanian Republic 2004). The service network in communities is inadequate and does not meet the needs of the families taking care of relatives with dementia (Government of Lithuanian Republic 2004). When families do not want to place older people with dementia into any of the care homes available, there are very limited services provided at home by formal caregivers. On the other hand, some relatively independent older people apply for permanent social care at institutions due to low availability of community-based services and low income.

Dependency levels could predict needs for services. Calculations under the Scottish model (Alzheimer Scotland 2000) estimate that 6 per cent of people with dementia would be independent, with care needed once a week for 11 per cent; care is needed at regular intervals during the day for dressing, meals and so on, for 48 per cent; and constant care and supervision is needed for the remaining 34 per cent. Using the Scottish model 39.3 per cent of all people with dementia would need institutional care, either in psychogeriatric wards, nursing homes, residential homes or other long stay facilities. The Scottish model is similar to that found by a Norwegian study (Engedal and Haugen 1993) which revealed that about 40 per cent of all people with dementia in Norway received institutional care.

Home-based care services

According to statistics collected by the European Commission there is a strong preference amongst EU governments and EU citizens alike for community-based care. Older people do not like to be institutionalized since often this leads to depersonalization and, in addition, institutional care is thought to be more costly compared to community-based care (Sutton 2000). According to the WHO, for low-income countries the most effective approach to service provision is to build community primary care services to support, educate and advise family caregivers, supplemented by subsidized home nursing or home care workers (WHO and WFN 2004, p.52).

In Lithuania, home-based services for older people are limited due to scarce resources, so priority is given to single people, with others left with limited opportunities to receive formal help. Those who need home help may apply to local municipally run social service departments. Older people are assessed for home help programmes based on social and medical criteria. In 2004, 3642 older people received some home-based help provided by social workers and visiting care workers (Department of Statistics of the Government of the Republic of Lithuania 2004). This equates to about 0.8 per cent of older people in Lithuania. By contrast, 8–24 per cent of Northern Europe's older citizens received home-based care.

In a study sample in London, people with dementia – 5.6 per cent of those receiving care – consumed 15.6 per cent of community care (Melzer *et al.* 2004). There is no data on prevalence of dementia among Lithuanian users of social services, but only people with mild dementia are eligible to receive home-based help. With changes in family structures due to new family living styles and decreased birth rates the numbers of older people living alone will increase. According to the Population Census, approximately 30 per cent of those older than 65 lived alone in 2001 (Government of Lithuanian Republic 2004). The risk of developing dementia is linked to age. There is therefore a considerable risk that people with dementia will be living alone. It means increased need for formal caregivers in the future. One of the priority areas of development of social services for older people in Lithuania is expansion of home-based care and non-stationary services. Currently about 47 per cent of all social care system clients receive permanent institutional care, and this type of care accounts for about 90 per cent of the budget allocated for social care services (Government of Lithuanian Republic 2004). Lack of community services can necessitate unnecessary use of acute hospital beds and accelerate transfers to long-term care facilities (Melzer *et al.* 2004), leading to increased costs for care. Community-based specialized services, such as day centres, home care and respite care, should be established and the use of assistive devices introduced into the care of people with dementia.

Another important issue persisting in the care of older people, and especially for people with dementia, in many European countries is the continued separation between social care and medical care. In Lithuania, the process of integration of health, nursing and social services is slow at both political and organizational levels (Government of Lithuanian Republic 2004). Greater integration and merged health and social services would ensure better quality of care, so that the needs of people with dementia and their families would be met more comprehensively.

Caregivers

'Worldwide, family caregivers are the cornerstone of support for people with dementia' (WHO and WFN 2004, p.52). They experience psychological, practical and economic strain. In resource-scarce settings, communities rely on family members alone to provide the care. In the majority of less developed countries informal caregivers are not supported by the state in a formal way, thus the burden of care is placed solely on caregivers. The combination of reduced family incomes and increased family expenditure is especially stressful in lower income countries (10/66 Dementia Research Group 2004). The traditions of extended families in less developed countries may alleviate the burden of caring, although principal caregivers are still under strain (Shaji *et al.* 2003). There are implications for the future as family units decrease in size and increasing numbers of older people live alone. There will be increasing demand for home help services even in the countries with extended families (Sutton 2000). Usually caregivers are in paid employment, and do not receive caregivers' allowances, although it is widely thought that 'when family members act as carers, this should be expressively recognized by giving them certain legal rights, and their own needs, for example, access to information, training, respite and other support services, should be fully met' (O'Shea and Group of Specialists on Improving the Quality of Life of Elderly Dependent Persons 2002, p.28).

Environment, staff and activities

Studies have suggested the efficiency of specific units and influence of adapted environments for people with dementia (Marshall 2001). Historically, the buildings and environment in health care and social care institutions were designed to meet architectural and hygiene requirements. There is still not enough attention paid to the environment in compensating for memory impairment, although with the concept of therapeutic environment greater attention is paid to compensating for disabilities not only for people with physical disability but also for those with cognitive impairment. In resource-scarce settings adaptation of the environment is less likely since investment in old buildings is costly and the effectiveness of adaptations can only be seen later. Investment in staff as part of a dementia-specific environment could have more instant effects. It is clear that purpose-built institutions for older people, including those with dementia, should be adapted to residents' needs.

People with dementia have many different needs, and different specialists and care professionals are required to meet these needs. According to the recommendations of the European Committee for Social Cohesion (O'Shea and Group of Specialists on Improving the Quality of Life of Elderly Dependent Persons 2002, p.26), 'people with dementia should receive dementia-specific services in appropriately designed environments from people who are trained to deliver such care'. The problem in less developed countries is two-fold: lack of specialists and staff in numbers and lack of formal training for those taking care of people with dementia. A Lithuanian study undertaken in a nursing hospital taking care of people with dementia revealed that there was a big demand for staff training on specific issues of dementia (Geduškaitė 2005). Lithuania has few occupational therapists or geriatricians. At the moment, there are 27 geriatricians in clinical practice, although according to demographic indicators and drawing on the experience of Western European countries, Lithuania needs approximately 100 geriatricians (Government of Lithuanian Republic 2004).

One of the main indicators of good quality social and health care services is the ratio of institutional staff to residents or clients. For people with moderate and severe dementia, staffing ratios of one nurse per two residents on all shifts is recommended (Eek *et al.* 1999). In resource-scarce settings this ratio could be difficult to achieve. Lack of staff in institutions produces problems of the adequacy of care and activity for people with dementia.

Meeting the psychosocial needs of persons with dementia remains a challenge (Innes and Surr 2001), and it is an even greater challenge to provide good care within tight budgets and often with workforces that have little or no formal training (Ballard *et al.* 2001). Basic physiological needs and life-threatening situations for people with dementia might be met, but more specific needs might be considered as side issues not requiring intervention. Many staff may still believe that people with dementia are unaware of the world and unable to benefit from interaction, and that they need just to be clean, warm and comfortable (Marshall 2001). Low staff–resident (or patient) ratios result in burn-out and staff who mechanistically provide basic care. Training and education of staff working with older people is a key element in ensuring quality of care, although investment in the environment in which care is provided is equally important. In under-resourced situations these key principles are affected adversely.

Policy and economics

In the majority of countries, policy for people with dementia is covered by policies regarding health and social welfare for older people and people with mental disorders, and welfare services are provided by national, state and local governments and by various private organizations. That said, in some less developed countries no national programme of care for older people exists or has been financed. No EU member states target significant resources specifically at services for Alzheimer's disease; the majority of provision is through generic services either at the primary care/community level, or through more specialized services for older people or mentally frail older people (Warner *et al.* 2002). Despite great differences in health and social care systems, service organization, cultural changes, financing and available resources the key principle embraced by all countries across different continents is the importance of and preference for home-based care and development of services in the community.

Economic evaluation allows policy makers, managers and clinicians to make choices that make optimum use of limited resources (Shah, Murthy and Suh 2002). Thus, economic evaluation becomes very important in countries and situations where allocation of resources to certain fields is limited. According to economic studies performed by other more developed countries dementia care is a high economic burden, and there is a great pressure on resources side-by-side with increasing demand for better quality of life (Warner *et al.* 2002). The most costly elements of care for people with dementia are the direct cost of institutionalization and the indirect cost of informal caregivers (Shah *et al.* 2002).

There are no health-economic studies in geriatric psychiatry from less developed countries, although some cost-effectiveness studies are published. In their review article Shah *et al.* (2002) indicate a number of reasons for the absence of economic studies in mental health and psychiatry from less developed countries. These included: lack of health economists and absence of training in this emerging discipline, mental health being a low priority health issue with less developed services, and data sets needed for economic analysis not being readily available (Shah *et al.* 2002). Extrapolation of economic studies from other countries may be inaccurate or sometimes even not possible due to different prevalence and incidence of diseases, different economic, health and social care service systems, lifestyles, cultures, attitudes, and other factors. That said, it is possible to adapt the methodology of economic evaluation successfully to local situations, health and social care systems although it should be noted that 'dementia care requirements should determine funding rather than have funding determining care needs' (O'Shea and O'Reilly 1999, p.67).

Evaluation

Scarce resources to diagnose, treat and provide adequate services to people with dementia impede the evaluation process itself. In dementia care, evaluations help to promote the value of services to users and to develop best practice (Parker 1999). Scarce resources may negatively affect the establishment of monitoring processes covering the whole system, limit the range of objectives to be evaluated and worsen quality of services in this way. The evaluation process itself is more complicated, since services are fragmented and belong to different systems (health and social care), and criteria are not the same. In countries with undeveloped dementia care and services, preference is given to establishing services and meeting the basic needs of service users and their families. On the other hand, newly set up health and social care services and institutions have to meet existing criteria in the countries (architectural, hygiene, and so on). Issuing a licence to state or private institutions to perform certain activities where they meet specified criteria is a part of evaluation processes. Internal control processes to ensure minimum standards are usually part of institutional policies. Shaw (2001) indicates that a number of external mechanisms exist to assure and improve the quality of health care, including the models of the International Organization for Standardization, the Baldrige criteria, peer review, accreditation, and registration and licensing. Shaw (2001, p.852) suggest that in addition to these mechanisms 'the organizations themselves should work towards a common set of standards, coordinate their activities'.

With increasing provision and development of specific services, the concept of quality of care becomes a practical issue to be applied in day-to-day life. Externally set standards, expectations, resources and training are all important in improving care (Chris and Chris 2001). It is suggested that minimum standards for institutions caring for people with dementia should be established in all countries where such information does not already guide care service provision.

In Lithuania, there is no integrated system for the evaluation of the health care and social service needs of older people. Major efforts are concentrated on development of health and social care services, and monitoring systems are not adequately established. Regular assessments are being carried out in state health care institutions and permanent social care institutions. The purpose of these evaluations is to find out whether the activities of institutions conform to requirements established in Lithuanian law.

The Department of Audit and Supervision of Social Establishments in Lithuania evaluates social care homes and homes for mentally ill persons, with monitoring systems following instructions which are mandatory for the state institutions and recommended for non-governmental and other types of institutions. These institutions must have an approved rulebook for staff, a rulebook for residents and be authorized by a public health centre; that is, have a passport of hygiene certifying that their premises meet the minimum hygiene requirements. The laws regulating institutional practice focus mainly on physical environment and basic functioning (Minister of Social Security and Labour 2002).

Assessment carried out among state social care institutions of Lithuania in 2003 revealed inconsistencies in the application of legal requirements: incorrect documentation and inappropriate staff structures, inadequate living environments and insufficient adaptation for disabled residents, and poor quality of services provided to the residents (Ministry of Social Security and Labour 2004). The Department of Audit and Supervision of Social Establishments, with support provided by the World Health Bank through the 'Changing Minds, Policies and Lives' project, developed a tool for measuring the quality of care in children's and adolescents' care institutions. The monitoring system and evaluation tools for basic functioning and quality of care in social care institutions for older people and mentally ill people will be developed based on these quality standards.

By evaluating only the basic criteria for functioning, the well-being of the residents can easily be overlooked. People with dementia need certain specialized services, but they also need compassion, understanding of their needs, appropriate activities, and human interaction (Scott 2001). Attitudes towards evaluation have to be shifted from evaluation of the physical environment and basic criteria to measurement of service user and resident well-being and the impact of the services. How this may be achieved in resource-scarce situations is problematic, but the process could begin by implementing minimum quality of care standards with regular monitoring. The listing of minimum requirements and the system of issuing of licences to institutions will help to ensure the basic quality of services for older people.

Service users – people with dementia – are very often left aside when service providers are planning services and standards. It should not be assumed that people with dementia cannot express their views on the quality of the care they receive. Recent research suggests that they can. In particular service users place very high importance on personal relationships with care staff (Mozley *et al.* 1999). In resource-scarce situations when prioritizing and planning service provision, conducting research and evaluating services the views of people with dementia should be included in parallel with the views of service providers and policy makers. Evaluation of dementia care is a part of research and studies are conducted in nearly all countries; only the extent and number of studies differ depending on allocation of resources, priorities and provision. In countries with undeveloped services for people suffering from dementia research and explorative studies play an important role in revealing the need for further intervention to improve the quality of care.

Future directions

New policies and laws designed for people with dementia and their caregivers will assist the development of services and alleviate the burden on informal caregivers. Incorporating models of economic evaluation and standards of quality of care in parallel with the development of services will contribute to building adequate levels of health and social care services. The development of new dementia-specific services is a necessity in countries with scarce services. One key dimension in future development of services is a focus on home-based care, integrated social health services, and community resources with particular support for informal caregivers. Education and training of formal and informal caregivers is one of the priority areas in enabling rapid positive results in the quality of care to be achieved. Regular and formal evaluation of the care of people with dementia with established, state-approved methods would provide valuable information, foster quality of care and help improve the quality of life of people with dementia. Undoubtedly, initial epidemiological studies on the prevalence and incidence of the disorder have to be conducted. These would reveal the extent of needs for health and social care services and assist in the appropriate allocation of resources.

Conclusion

Lack of data on prevalence and incidence of dementia impedes the assessment of needs for and the evaluation of future developments in health and social care services. Timely evaluation of needs would encourage adequate resource utilization. In resource-scarce situations, health and social care services for people with dementia are fragmented and informal caregivers are faced with a dearth of formal support. More attention should be paid to the development of home-based care, the provision of dementia-specific units in long-term care institutions, and co-operation within and between health care and social care sectors. Mandatory, systematic monitoring of services and systems of care, which is currently incomplete or non-existent in some countries, should be developed in parallel with the expansion of high-quality care services.

References

10/66 Dementia Research Group (2004) 'Care arrangements for people with dementia in developing countries.' *International Journal of Geriatric Psychiatry 19*, 170–177.

Alvarado-Esquil, C., Hernandez-Alvarado, A.B., Tapia-Rodriguez, R.O., Guerrero-Iturbe, A., Rodriguez-Corral, K. and Martinez, S.E. (2004) 'Prevalence of dementia and Alzheimer's disease in elders of nursing homes and a senior center of Durango City, Mexico.' *BMC Psychiatry 4*, 3. Available from www.biomedcentral.com/1471-244X/4/3.

Alzheimer Scotland (2000) *Planning Signposts for Dementia Care Services.* Edinburgh: Alzheimer Scotland.

Ballard, C., Fossey, J., Chithramohan, R., Howard, R., Burns, A., Thompson, P., Tadros, G. and Fairbairn, A. (2001) 'Quality of care in private sector and NHS facilities for people with dementia: cross sectional survey.' *British Medical Journal 323*, 426–427.

Berr, C., Wancata, J. and Ritchie, K. (2005) 'Prevalence of dementia in the elderly of Europe.' *European Neuropsychopharmacology 15*, 463–471.

Breteler, M.M., Ott, A. and Hofman, A. (1998) 'The new epidemic: frequency of dementia in the Rotterdam Study.' *Haemostasis 3–4*, 117–123.

Burns, A., O'Brien, J. and Ames, D. (eds) (2005) *Dementia.* London: Hodder Arnold.

Chris, E. and Chris, F. (2001) 'Dementia care mapping is an inadequate tool for research.' *British Medical Journal 323*, 1427.

Davidoniene, O. (2005) Personal communication.

de Exter, A., Hermans, H., Dosijak, M. and Busse, R. (2004) *Health Care Systems in Transition: The Netherlands.* Copenhagen: WHO Regional Office for Europe on behalf of the European Observatory on Health Systems and Policies.

Department of Audit and Supervision of Social Establishments at the Ministry of Social Security and Labour (2005) *The Report on First Half-year of 2005.* (Socialiniu istaigu prieáiuros ir audito departamentas prie Socialines apsaugos ir darbo ministerijos, 2005 m. I pusmecio ataskaita.) Available from www.sipad.lt//customfiles/lt/2005 _I_pusmecio_1.doc

Department of Statistics of the Government of the Republic of Lithuania (2004) Health and Social Care. Available from www.std.lt/uploads/1127300801_Socialines_ paslaugos_2004.doc.

Department of Statistics of the Government of the Republic of Lithuania (2005) Population and social statistics. Available from www.std.lt/en/pages/view/?id =1385.

Eek, A., Engedal, K., Holthe, T., Nygard, A.M. and Oksengaard, A.R. (1999) *Care for People with Dementia in Norway.* Oslo: The Norwegian Centre for Dementia Research.

Engedal, K. and Haugen, P.K. (1993) 'The prevalence of dementia in a sample of elderly Norwegians.' *International Geriatric Psychiatry 8*, 565–570.

EUROSTAT (2005) Available from http://ec.europa.eu/comm.eurostat/.

Ferri, C., Prince, M., Brayne, C., Brodaty, H., Fratiglioni, L., Ganguli, M., Hall, K., Hasegawa, K., Hendrie, H., Huang, Y., Jorm, A., Mathers, C., Menezes, P., Rimmer, E. and Scazufca, M. (2005) 'Global prevalence of dementia: a Delphi consensus study.' *The Lancet 366*, 2112–2117.

Fratiglioni, L., Grut, M., Forsell, Y., Viitanen, M., Grafstrøm, M., Holmen, K., Ericsson, K., Backman, L., Ahlbom, A. and Winblad, B. (1991) 'Prevalence of Alzheimer's disease and other dementias in an elderly urban population: relationship with age, sex, and education.' *Neurology 41*, 1886–1892.

Geduškaitė, L. (2005) 'Kauno K.Griniaus slaugos ir palaikomojo gydymo ligonines veiklos optimizavimas pritaikant demencija serganciu pacientu slaugai.' Public Health Masters thesis, Kaunas University of Medicine, Kaunas.

Government of Lithuanian Republic (2004) The National Strategy of Overcoming Consequences of Aging Population (Nacionalines gyventoju senejimo paskemiu iveikimo srategija) 2004 m. biráelio 14 d. Nr. 737, Vilnius.

Innes, A. and Surr, C. (2001) 'Measuring the well-being of people with dementia living in formal care settings: the use of Dementia Care Mapping.' *Aging and Mental Health 5*, 3, 258–268.

Jha, S. and Patel, R. (2004) 'Some observations on the spectrum of dementia.' *Neurology India 52*, 213–214.

Kinsella, K. and Velkoff, V.A. (2001) *An Ageing World: 2001. International Population Records.* Washington DC: US Department of Health and Human Services, US Census Bureau.

Knapp, M. (1995) 'Resource scarcity chasing scarce resources: health economics and geriatric psychiatry.' *International Journal of Geriatric Psychiatry 10*, 821–829.

Macijauskiene, J. and Engedal, K. (2005) 'Medicosocial care for persons suffering from Alzheimer's disease and related disorders.' *Medicina 41*, 67–72.

Marshall, M. (2001) 'The challenge of looking after people with dementia.' *British Medical Journal 323*, 410–411.

Melzer, D., Pearce, K., Cooper, B. and Brayne, C. (2004) 'Alzheimer's disease and other dementias.' In A. Stevens, J. Raftery, J. Mant and S. Simpson (eds) *Health Care Needs Assessment: The Epidemiologically Based Needs Assessment Reviews – First Series Update*. Abingdon: Radcliffe Medical Press.

Minister of Social Security and Labour (2002) Order No 97 of 9 July 2002 on Approval of the Requirements for Stationary Institutions of Social Care and the Procedure for Referring Individuals to Inpatient Institutions of Social Care, Valstybes áinios (Official Gazette), 2002, No. 76–3274.

Ministry of Social Security and Labour (2004) *Social Report 2003*. Vilnius: Ministry of Social Security and Labour.

Mozley, C., Huxley, P., Sutcliffe, C., Bagley, H., Burns, A., Challis, D. and Cordingley, L. (1999) '"Not knowing where I am doesn't mean I don't know what I like": cognitive impairment and quality of life responses in elderly people.' *International Journal of Geriatric Psychiatry 14*, 776–783.

O'Brien, J.A. and Caro, J.J. (2001) 'Alzheimer's disease and other dementia in nursing homes: levels of management and cost.' *International Psychogeriatrics 13*, 347–358.

OECD Health Data (2004) First edition, WHO Regional Office for Europe. Available from www.czso.cz/eng/redakce.nsf/i/34FEAE9FA60FFFA7C1256F10003F4A 0F/$File/International_comp.pdf.

O'Shea, E. and Group of Specialists on Improving the Quality of Life of Elderly Dependent Persons (2002) *Improving the Quality of Life of Elderly Persons in Situations of Dependency*. Strasbourg: Council of Europe Publishing.

O'Shea, E. and O'Reilly, S. (1999) *An Action Plan on Dementia*. Dublin: National Council on Ageing and Older People.

Ott, A., Breteler, M.M., van Harskamp, F., Claus, J.J., van der Cammen, T.J.M., Grobbee, D.E. and Hofman, A. (1995) 'Prevalence of Alzheimer's disease and vascular dementia: association with education. The Rotterdam study.' *British Medical Journal 310*, 970–973.

Parker, J. (1999) 'Education and learning for the evaluation of dementia care: the perceptions of social workers in training.' *Education and Ageing 14*, 3, 297–314.

Puras, D., Germanavicius, A., Povilaitis, R., Veniute, M. and Jasilionis, D. (2004) 'Lithuania mental health country profile.' *International Review of Psychiatry 16*, 117–125.

Scott, J. (2001) 'Quality of care for people with dementia.' *British Medical Journal 323*, 1427.

Shah, A., Murthy, S. and Suh, G.K. (2002) 'Is mental health economics important in geriatric psychiatry in developing countries?' *International Journal of Geriatric Psychiatry 17*, 758–764.

Shaji, K.S., Smitha, K., Praveen Lal, K. and Prince, M. (2003) 'Caregivers of people with Alzheimer's disease: a qualitative study from the Indian 10/66 Dementia Research Network.' *International Journal of Geriatric Psychiatry 18*, 1–6.

Shaw, Ch. (2001) 'External assessment of health care.' *British Medical Journal 322*, 851–854.

Suh, G.H. and Shah, A. (2001) 'A review of the epidemiological transition in dementia – cross-national comparisons of the indices related to Alzheimer's disease and vascular dementia.' *Acta Psychiatrica Scandinavica 104*, 4–11.

Sutton, A. (2000) 'Old age and the economy.' *Catholic Medical Quarterly 288*, 19–24.

Warner, M., Furnish, S., Longley, M. and Lawlor, B. (eds) (2002) *Alzheimer's Disease: Policy and Practice across Europe.* Oxford: Radcliffe Medical Press.

WHO (2005) Mental Health Atlas. Available from www.who.int.

WHO and WFN (2004) Atlas: Country Resources for Neurological Disorders. Geneva: WHO. Available from www.who.int/mental_health/neurogy/neurology_atlas_lr.pdf.

WHO Statistical Information System (WHOSIS) (2002) Country Health Indicators. Available from www3.who.int/whosis/country/indicators.cfm.

Chapter 14

Building on the Lessons of Evaluations

Louise McCabe and Anthea Innes

This chapter discusses key challenges facing those concerned with evaluating dementia care in the future. The preceding chapters have provided interesting insights into how such challenges can be overcome. The book highlights issues requiring considerable energy from the evaluator to ensure that evaluations can meet the objectives of the commissioner while ensuring that the views of key stakeholders are heard. It is important that recommendations for future action can be used by stakeholders to develop dementia care in the future.

Building from the lessons of others involved in evaluation this chapter begins by exploring four practical challenges that remain for those who take on an evaluation:

- working ethically
- ensuring the service user's voice is heard
- the costs of evaluating
- how to choose the right evaluation design.

The second part of this chapter considers a broader challenge; that is, to make sense of it all. By this we mean, what are the aims of dementia care and how does the process of evaluation fit within these? How does the practice of evaluation relate to broader social issues such as the policy context and our understanding of dementia and dementia care? Further to that, how does evaluation take place in a world of competing priorities and scarce resources? Finally, we explore the different aims of evaluations, for example do they aim to demonstrate that a service is good or aim to improve care, to meet government policies or perhaps to appeal to the ongoing movement of hearing users' views? This chapter addresses this complexity and poses questions for future evaluators.

Remaining challenges
Working ethically

Ethical practice when conducting evaluations that involve people with dementia is paramount; people with dementia are often vulnerable due to their dependence on others. Several of the authors of preceding chapters raise important points relating to evaluating ethically. Kirkevold highlights the importance of ethical practice by staff and caregivers as well as the researchers involved in evaluation. Indeed ethical practice is something everyone should be concerned with. Christie offers us a detailed and incisive exploration of the issues around ethical practice and evaluation. She emphasizes the importance of not seeing ethics as one stage of an evaluation but stresses that it should be considered at each stage and should be an ongoing process. Her advice concerning ethics boards is to see them as a useful and important stage in the research design to reflect upon the design of the evaluation and its ethical implications rather than a hurdle to be negotiated. Several of the authors raise the issues of consent and competency. This is an area that continues to produce debate and imaginative methods are needed to ensure that people with dementia are encouraged to take part in the consent process rather than carers or professionals. Consent involves the provision of information, the capacity to understand it and the voluntary nature of agreed participation (Medical Research Council 1991).

Bowes, in her discussion on technology, highlights new ethical dilemmas associated with new types of care and support being offered to people with dementia. Technology offers new solutions to providing care for people with dementia but also brings new challenges for ethical practice. The example of electronic tagging is a case in point.

Ensuring the service user's voice is heard

Policy rhetoric such as that found in the Green Paper *Independence, Well-being and Choice, Our Vision for the Future of Social Care for Adults in England* (Department of Health 2005) supports including service users and providing individualized care plans. Services are slowly changing to reflect this and service users are increasingly involved in decisions about their care and support. It is also important to include service users in any evaluations of services or support that they receive.

It seems clear that the involvement of people with dementia in evaluation processes is a practice that is receiving increasing attention and is being undertaken more often (Wilkinson 2002). The policy background, as discussed by McCabe, reflects a growing interest in the views of service users and people with dementia. It is possible to involve people with dementia in the evaluation process but their involvement needs to be handled sensitively if it is to be effective. Murphy shares his experience of involving people with dementia in evaluation processes and offers a seven-point checklist of approaches to involving people with dementia. This checklist includes suggestions such as: establish a relationship with the person; view the interaction more as a conversation than an interview; and maximize the 'immediacy' of what is being evaluated. He highlights the challenges to involving people with dementia and raises the importance of issues such as consent, intruding into people's lives and the expectations which service users and their carers may have about being involved in research. Christie in her discussion on ethical practice also raises important issues for consideration when involving people with dementia and discusses the process of gaining consent, concluding that an ongoing consent process should be adopted (Reid, Ryan and Enderby 2001). Both chapters identify that involving people with dementia may be a difficult and time-consuming process but it is an important process that should be undertaken.

In her discussion on external and internal evaluation Lechner raises important points about insiders and outsiders and the benefits and limitations of each approach. People with dementia are in effect the most internal type of evaluator and including people with dementia in evaluations will add all the advantages seen when using internal evaluators.

It is clear that involving people with dementia in evaluations is a desirable practice but it may not be an easy thing to achieve. In order to involve people with dementia they need to be recruited, agree to take part and then be enabled to undertake their given role.

Tyrrell discusses the problems encountered when recruiting people with dementia to take part in an evaluation of their experiences of choice. Often the people with dementia who do take part in research are the individuals who are already being supported to express their own views and maintain control in their lives. In addition, evaluators often work with gatekeepers such as physicians or care home managers and they may be the ones who 'select' participants for research. It may be more valuable to hear the voices of people with dementia who are more marginalized or seen as 'unsuitable' for research but this group is difficult to access.

Once participants are recruited then it is necessary to gain their consent to participate and ensure that this consent remains throughout the evaluation process. This issue was discussed throughout preceding chapters and needs careful consideration and innovative approaches to achieve this.

However, it is not enough just to include people with dementia in evaluations; their voices must also be heard. Murphy cautions against tokenism in research whereby people with dementia are included but no real attention is paid to their views which are, therefore, not subsequently implemented. Murphy emphasizes the need to hear the voices of people with dementia as they provide a unique and crucial viewpoint of the service or intervention being evaluated.

People with dementia who do take part in research (for example, McKillop 2002; Robinson 2002) often report positive outcomes in terms of feeling included and having an impact on services. McKillop (2002) does, however, raise the point that interview questions may be intrusive and mean revisiting difficult memories. Including people with dementia is a vital part of any evaluation and this process should be approached with sensitivity and careful thought.

Service evaluations such as inspections, which are closely related to policy, do attempt to include people with dementia in the evaluation process. Inspectors may discuss the care service with service users during an inspection process. However, the way in which these views are incorporated into any future service development is seldom clear.

This section has discussed the importance of hearing the voices of people with dementia in evaluations. It is also important to remember to include the viewpoints of other stakeholders within the service or intervention such as family carers and frontline staff; both these groups may be marginalized in evaluations.

The costs of evaluating

Macijauskiene among others raises the issue of resources for evaluation. In less developed countries resources will be scarce for the provision of dementia care so obtaining additional resources to undertake evaluations may be more difficult. The resource implications of evaluating dementia care in more developed countries may also be related to financial resources. Service providers and commissioners may not see the value of different types of evaluations. The policy-driven and compulsory evaluation processes described by McCabe are relatively cost-effective and allow all care services to be evaluated in some way. As discussed these evaluations have many flaws both methodologically and in the reports produced as outcomes. However, they are often the only type of evaluation a care service will receive; this is particularly true in resource-limited situations such as those found in less developed countries.

The expense of an in-depth qualitative evaluation will often be prohibitory but, as the chapters in this book illustrate, for example Chapter 8, the information and outcomes from these will be valuable. These types of evaluation are not just financially costly but also require time commitments from different stakeholders for example care staff may find it difficult to find time to take part in interviews or complete questionnaires.

How to choose the right evaluation design

As raised in Chapter 1 and addressed by various authors through the book, the key question to ask at the start of an evaluation is – what methods are most appropriate to the question we are seeking to answer?

The chapters in this book present a wide range of approaches to evaluation in dementia care. These range from quantitative, experimental type processes (for example, see Chapter 7) through to qualitative and more alternative methods (for example, see Chapter 8). When designing an evaluation it is necessary to choose methods appropriate to the task at hand. The purpose of the evaluation and the intended outcomes should be considered when designing the evaluation as well as consideration of the different participants and stakeholders.

As Cantley cautions, the experimental approach may be favoured by some, particularly by medical professionals, but it is difficult to achieve in complex social settings. Gibson, Haight and Michel describe a quasi-experimental approach to evaluating a reminiscence intervention for people with dementia. Their chapter shows that with innovative thought and careful planning it is possible to implement rigorous 'experimental' research and produce useful and convincing evidence. Their discussion illustrates the need to involve different stakeholders in the evaluation process and the complexity of the process. They also highlight the fact that care situations are very complex and it is often difficult to assess accurately the impact of a specific intervention when there are so many other variables present in a given situation. Wijk also discusses the use of quasi-experimental approaches to evaluating the impact of environmental factors and recommends this type of approach for evaluating environmental factors such as colour, sound and lighting. Wijk's chapter illustrates the breadt h of different approaches used to evaluate the impact of the environment for people with dementia. This is an area where an increasing amount of research is being undertaken and offers examples of innovative approaches.

These types of experimentalist approach often focus on measurable outcomes. As care cultures become increasingly target-oriented, evidence-based outcomes are becoming more important to a range of stakeholders, including commissioners and service providers as well as service users themselves. Gibson, Haight and Michel describe the use of a range of outcome measures, which they use to assess the impact of a reminiscence-based intervention. The range of measures they use helps to provide a detailed and clear picture of the outcomes of the intervention.

The differences found between different outcome measures illustrate the need to take a broad approach when considering outcomes as it can be difficult to identify specific outcomes for people with dementia.

Other chapters, for example those by Kirkevold, Tyrrell, and Innes and Kelly, describe approaches to evaluation which do not follow an experimentalist approach and as such avoid the pressure felt by dementia practitioners to fit with widely accepted experimentalist approaches. These chapters identify and describe alternative and innovative approaches to evaluating dementia care services and interventions. Innes and Kelly explore the use of DCM in long stay services and discuss its advantages and limitations. Within their chapter they discuss a 'tool box' approach to evaluation, suggesting that a range of approaches to evaluation are needed to produce valuable and rigorous results. A combination of DCM, audit tools and ethnographic measures are used to evaluate long stay care settings.

In addition to choosing the right tools for each evaluation there are practical challenges in carrying out the evaluation. The preceding chapters illustrate many of the practical challenges to undertaking evaluations. Policy-driven evaluations, as described by McCabe, pose practical challenges related to the nature of the evaluation processes they involve: they should be standardized, achievable within time and resource constraints, include a range of views and be easily reportable and accessible. These practical considerations limit the potential of these evaluation processes and constrain the outcomes from them. It is difficult to produce one method that can be used across a range of services and that will effectively evaluate them.

Kirkevold's discussion of evaluating the practice of covert medication administration illustrates some other practical problems in evaluation. This practice is often hidden and under-reported; therefore a sensitive approach is required to evaluate the practice. Kirkevold discusses the ways in which these practices can be brought out into the open and be evaluated and assessed in a balanced and useful manner.

Practical challenges may appear to be overcome when evaluating the use of technology due to the built-in ability for technology to record what is happening (for example, fall detectors recording number of falls). It is important, however, to fully understand the implications of what the technology has recorded and to investigate further what is really happening.

Approaches to evaluation in dementia care should, where possible, employ appropriate and individual methodologies designed to meet the specific purpose of each evaluation. Throughout the book there has been a strong recommendation for the use of mixed or multiple methods for effective evaluation. A flexible approach to the practicalities of evaluation is needed to ensure that evaluation outcomes are beneficial to different stakeholders.

Evaluation in dementia care

This section considers the following questions. What are the aims of dementia care and how does the process of evaluation fit within these? How does the practice of evaluation relate to broader social issues such as the policy context and our understanding of dementia and dementia care? How does evaluation take place in a world of competing priorities and scarce resources?

Over the past ten years many changes have taken place both in the way dementia is understood and conceptualized and in the ways people with dementia are cared for. Advances in medical knowledge have led to earlier diagnosis and new treatment options. The lower age of people being diagnosed and new treatment options are influencing perceptions of the condition. The concept of person-centred care (Kitwood 1997) is now common parlance among dementia practitioners although there may not be a clear definition of what this means for specific care practice situations (Innes, Macpherson and McCabe 2006). It is now more widely accepted that people with dementia do not have to live limited lives within residential or nursing institutions and that quality care can improve the quality of life for a person with dementia and improve their symptoms (Downs 2000; Marshall 2005). A wider range of care services are now available and innovative approaches to long-term care are being developed.

In the UK, as in other countries, these changes have been influenced by changing health and social policy. The National Health Service and Community Care Act 1990 introduced notions of user empowerment and choice of services for service users. This Act also encouraged the growth of a mixed economy of care; the gradual withdrawal of responsibility for the provision of care from local authorities and the encouragement of private and voluntary organizations has led to an increase in specialist services designed for people with dementia. Specific services have embraced concepts such as person-centred care and aim to provide services their users want. New advances in technology and design are also influencing the types of care service available for people with dementia.

There is an underlying theme to these policy and service changes of user empowerment and choice – hearing the voice of people with dementia. Dementia care now has the aim of providing good quality care that suits the needs of each individual and evaluation of services is a key way in which this can be achieved. The process of evaluation therefore becomes central in facilitating policy makers, commissioners, practitioners, frontline workers and carers in understanding the views of people with dementia. The following discussion highlights the impact of ongoing changes in diagnosis and in service provision.

As Tyrrell highlights, early diagnosis means that many more people with dementia are now aware of their diagnosis and are in a stronger position to influence the care provided to them. Early diagnosis means that people with dementia are able to plan for their future and make choices about the kind of care they wish to receive. In order to make these choices and influence care practice people with dementia need to be involved in evaluations of dementia care/support. The pervasive ageism in western cultures disempowers older people and devalues their views; people with dementia are particularly vulnerable to this type of discrimination. If people with dementia are diagnosed sooner, at a younger age, their voices are perhaps more likely to be heard. Several younger people with dementia including James McKillop and Lynn Jackson, and groups such as the Scottish Dementia Working group (www.alzscot.org/pages/sdwg.htm), are increasingly making their voices heard and campaigning for people with dementia.

In the UK ongoing policy changes have led to an increase in services provided by private and voluntary organizations and increasing joint working between health and social care providers. People with dementia

receive multi-disciplinary care and support. This makes evaluation processes more complex. In addition other professionals such as engineers
working with technology and architects designing care facilities are now
becoming involved in different ways in dementia care (for example, Wijk
in progress).

Care environments are changing and becoming more sophisticated as
illustrated by Wijk in her discussions of care environments and Bowes in
her discussion of technology. There has been increasing investment in
assistive technology with the aim of supporting people at home, improving their quality of life and cutting hospital admissions with the ultimate
aim of reducing costs. New technology brings new challenges to ethical
practice as highlighted above and it also adds new aspects to evaluation
processes. This complexity in service design and provision makes evaluation even more important.

Resource implications

When resources are limited the importance of in-depth evaluation may not
be emphasized or indeed possible. Macijauskiene discusses the scarcity of
resources in less developed countries where basic inspections of services
may be the only type of evaluation possible. Competing priorities for
service providers may limit their ability to participate in or commission
evaluations. Bowes, however, reminds us that evaluations may be used as a
method to reduce costs. Evaluating new technologies may have the
purpose of investigating how these new approaches to care may be more
economical in the longer term. Service providers may also be asked to
produce evidence of their cost-effectiveness and evaluation may be the
way to do this.

The different aims of evaluations

A clear understanding of the purpose of the evaluation is needed when
planning the design of the project. It is important to consider the audience
of the report and/or the outcomes of evaluation. Is the evaluation intended
to lead to practical changes to the service or intervention? For example,
local authority inspection teams have clearly stated aims including that of

improving services; they are also backed up by the legislation to impose changes to services. The aim of these types of evaluation may also include meeting government priorities. Other possible aims include demonstrating the service is good for users or perhaps cost-effective for funders and commissioners. Another reason might be to appeal to the movement to hear user views. All of these aims along with consideration of stakeholders and outcomes will influence the design of the evaluation and the choice of methods.

It is not enough just to evaluate services for people with dementia; it is also important to evaluate practices such as that of administering medication (as discussed by Kirkevold) and the experiences people with dementia have in health and social care settings (such as the experiences of choice described by Tyrrell).

Future implications for evaluators

Care provision for people with dementia is a field that is constantly changing and developing. Good evaluations can help to drive this process in the right direction and ensure the voices of people with dementia are heard. In conclusion four future challenges for evaluators are:

- to give careful consideration to the ethical implications for all stakeholders

- to truly listen to the voices of people with dementia and incorporate their views in any evaluation outcomes

- to consider financial and other costs and the relationship between evaluations and resources

- to choose the right design for each evaluation dependent on the aims of the evaluation and the desired outcomes.

References
Department of Health (2005) *Independence, Well-being and Choice, Our Vision for the Future of Social Care for Adults in England.* London: HMSO. Available at: www.dh.gov.uk/asset Root/ 04/10/64/78/04106478.pdf.

Downs, M. (2000) 'Dementia in a social-cultural context: an idea whose time has come.' *Ageing and Society 20*, 3, 369–373.

Innes, I., Macpherson, S. and McCabe, L. (2006) *Promoting Person Centred Care at the Frontline.* York: Joseph Rowntree Foundation. Available at: www.jrf.org.uk/book shop/eBooks/9781859354520.pdf.

Kitwood, T. (1997) *Dementia Reconsidered: The Person Comes First.* Buckingham: Open University Press.

McKillop, J. (2002) 'Did research alter anything?' In H. Wilkinson (ed.) *The Perspectives of People with Dementia: Research Methods and Motivations.* London: Jessica Kingsley Publishers.

Marshall, M. (2005) 'Perspectives on rehabilitation and dementia.' In M. Marshall (ed.) *Perspectives on Rehabilitation and Dementia.* London: Jessica Kingsley Publishers.

Medical Research Council (MRC) (1991) *The Ethical Conduct of Research on the Mentally Incapacitated.* London: MRC.

Reid, D., Ryan, T. and Enderby, P. (2001) 'What does it mean to listen to people with dementia?' *Disability and Society 16,* 3, 377–392.

Robinson, E. (2002) 'Should people with Alzheimer's disease take part in research?' In H. Wilkinson (ed.) *The Perspectives of People with Dementia: Research Methods and Motivations.* London: Jessica Kingsley Publishers.

Wijk, H. (in progress) 'Effects of adjustments of the physical environments for people with dementia.'

Wilkinson, H. (2002) 'Including people with dementia in research: methods and motivations.' In H. Wilkinson (ed.) *The Perspectives of People with Dementia: Research Methods and Motivations.* London: Jessica Kingsley Publishers.

Subject Index

Author Index